Epidemiology and Biostatistics

Bryan Kestenbaum

Epidemiology and Biostatistics

An Introduction to Clinical Research

Second Edition

Editors
Noel S. Weiss, MD PhD
Department of Epidemiology
University of Washington
Seattle, WA
USA

Abigail Shoben, PhD
Biostatistics, College of Public Health
The Ohio State University
Columbus, OH
USA

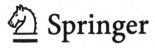 Springer

Bryan Kestenbaum, MD, MS
Division of Nephrology
Department of Medicine
University of Washington
Seattle, WA
USA

ISBN 978-3-319-96642-7   ISBN 978-3-319-96644-1   (eBook)
https://doi.org/10.1007/978-3-319-96644-1

Library of Congress Control Number: 2018955511

This Springer imprint is published by the registered company Springer Nature Switzerland AG
The registered company address is: Gewerbestrasse 11, 6330 Cham, Switzerland

Preface

This textbook was originally created from a disparate collection of materials used to teach Epidemiology and Biostatistics to second-year medical students at the University of Washington. These materials included handouts, practice problems, guides to reading journal articles, quizzes, notes from student help sessions, and student emails. The primary goal of these materials, and now this book, is to recreate the perspective of learning Epidemiology and Biostatistics for the first time. With critical editing assistance from Epidemiology faculty, graduate students in Epidemiology and Biostatistics, and the students themselves, I have tried to preserve the innate logic and connectedness of clinical research methods and demonstrate their application.

The textbook is intended to provide students with the tools necessary to form their own informed conclusions from research studies. More than ever, a clear understanding of the fundamental aspects of Epidemiology and Biostatistics is needed to successfully navigate the increasingly complex methods used by modern research studies. The appetite for studies of human health has grown at a rapid pace; yet, the interpretation of findings obtained from these studies has not always keep pace.

In this second edition, I have tried to further clarify concepts that are most difficult for students and provide a more logical structure to the material. Many new examples have been added throughout the textbook to reenforce these concepts.

This book could not have been created without the dedicated help of the editors, the teaching assistants, and most importantly the students, who asked the important questions. I would especially like to thank my family who patiently allowed me so much time to write.

Seattle, WA, USA   Bryan Kestenbaum, MD, MS

Contents

Part I
Epidemiology

Chapter 1
Causal Relationships in Health and Disease

Summary of Learning Points

1.1 Inferring causation in research studies is important for treating and preventing disease.

1.2 Criteria favoring causal inference in epidemiologic and clinical research include:

    1.2.1 Randomized evidence

    1.2.2 Strong associations

    1.2.3 Temporal association between exposure and outcome

    1.2.4 Exposure or dose varying association

    1.2.5 Biologic plausibility

In July of 1998, a 55-year-old man developed a new and unusual appearing rash on both arms. His symptoms began approximately 3 weeks earlier, when he first experienced weakness in his left hand. His physician ordered a magnetic resonance imaging (MRI) scan of the brain, which was normal. Suspecting that the man's symptoms were caused by a transient ischemic attack, or mini-stroke, his physician prescribed aspirin.

The man's left arm weakness resolved but was soon followed by the development of hardened plaques over the skin of his arms. A dermatologist, puzzled by this unusual rash, performed a skin biopsy, which revealed dense scarring and infiltrates of fibroblasts (cells involved in wound healing). The dermatologist and the primary physician were unable to find any previous reports in the medical literature that matched this man's unusual condtion.

The patient's medical history included end-stage kidney disease, for which he received dialysis 3 times per week. He also had high blood pressure, asthma, and gout. He had quit smoking 10 years ago and had not recently started any new medications except for the aspirin.

What could be causing this unusual condition?

Two years later, a report was published describing 15 people who developed hardened plaques over the skin of their arms and legs [1]. *Skin biopsies revealed*

© Springer Nature Switzerland AG 2019
B. Kestenbaum, *Epidemiology and Biostatistics*,
https://doi.org/10.1007/978-3-319-96644-1_1

diffuse scarring, similar to the findings of the patient described above. All of the people in this report were receiving dialysis for end-stage kidney disease. The condition was subsequently named "nephrogenic systemic fibrosis" or NSF.

The exclusive occurrence of this new condition among people with kidney disease suggests that the cause may be related to kidney failure or to the dialysis procedure itself. However, NSF had never been previously reported over decades of experience with dialysis. The new appearance of this illness suggests that some recently introduced risk factor, possibly connected with a specific geographic region or emerging practice pattern, might be the cause.

Over the next several years, additional cases of NSF were reported from the United States, Europe, Russia, and India. The condition was found exclusively among people with advanced kidney disease. In some instances, NSF progressed to include scarring of internal organs with up to 30% of affected people dying from the disease. No cause was identified.

Reports of NSF from around the world exclude an obvious geographic pattern to the condition. A useful next step would be to carefully scrutinize the characteristics of patients who developed NSF in attempt to identify patterns that might suggest a possible cause. Table 1.1 presents representative data from an initial report of ten patients who were diagnosed with NSF.

These data do not reveal an obvious pattern with respect to age, sex, or type of kidney disease among this group of NSF patients. The clinical presentation of NSF as a scarring skin lesion suggests that this condition could be caused by the accumulation of some harmful substance. Patients who undergo dialysis frequently receive intravenous iron to treat anemia (low red blood cell count). Moreover, dialysis leads to the retention of a protein called beta-2 microglobulin, which can build up in tissues. Table 1.2 describes patterns of intravenous iron use and circulating beta-2 microglobulin levels in another group of patients with NSF.

Six of these ten patients were receiving intravenous iron. This frequency appears to be high; however, appraisal of a possible link with the disease requires comparison with the frequency of intravenous iron use among otherwise similar people who do not have NSF. Approximately 65% of the general dialysis population (without

Table 1.1 Series of patients with nephrogenic systemic fibrosis

	Age	Sex	Cause of kidney disease
Patient 1	54	Male	Diabetes
Patient 2	68	Female	Glomerulonephritis
Patient 3	39	Female	Diabetes
Patient 4	32	Female	Polycystic kidney disease
Patient 5	76	Male	Renal vascular disease
Patient 6	57	Male	Diabetes
Patient 7	49	Female	Glomerulonephritis
Patient 8	53	Male	Hypertension
Patient 9	64	Female	Diabetes
Patient 10	67	Female	Renal vascular disease

Table 1.2 Second series of patients with nephrogenic systemic fibrosis

	Intravenous iron use	Serum beta-2 microglobulin
Patient 1	No	No
Patient 2	No	No
Patient 3	Yes	No
Patient 4	Yes	No
Patient 5	No	No
Patient 6	Yes	No
Patient 7	Yes	No
Patient 8	No	Yes
Patient 9	Yes	No
Patient 10	Yes	No

Table 1.3 Report of nephrogenic systemic fibrosis with magnetic resonance imaging (MRI)

	Recent contrast MRI study
Patient 1	Yes
Patient 2	Yes
Patient 3	Yes
Patient 4	Yes
Patient 5	Yes

NSF) typically receive intravenous iron, diminishing the likelihood that this agent is causing the disease. Only one patient with NSF in this report had detectable beta-2 microglobulin, suggesting that this protein is also not likely to be a cause of the illness.

An important breakthrough came in 2006, when researchers reviewed the medical records of five patients who had recently developed NSF to discover a previously unrecognized link with MRI procedures, shown in Table 1.3 [2].

All five people who developed NSF in this series had previously received an MRI procedure within 4 weeks before the onset of the disease. This intriguing finding suggests that MRI, or some characteristic associated with this procedure, could be the cause of NSF. However, these preliminary findings should be viewed with some degree of skepticism. The study evaluated only five people, raising the possibility of a chance association with MRI. Second, information regarding the frequency of MRI procedures among dialysis patients who do not develop NSF is needed for comparison. Third, MRI is used to diagnose a wide variety of medical conditions. It is possible that one or more of these conditions, and not the MRI procedure itself, is causing NSF.

What are next steps for investigating the possibility that MRI procedures are the cause of this illness? Subjecting people to MRI solely for the purpose of investigating NSF would be unethical, given the seriousness of this condition. An alternative approach would be to identify one group of dialysis patients who completed an MRI procedure for a clinical indication and a second group of dialysis patients who did not undergo an MRI. Such a study could then compare the occurrence of NSF among these groups. This approach would not be perfect. Characteristics of patients who received an MRI may differ from those of patients who did not undergo this procedure, distorting a potential association with NSF. Moreover, NSF is a rare illness, necessitating study of large numbers of patients to observe sufficient NSF cases for comparison. Nonetheless, such studies could be combined with supportive data from other types of studies to examine the root cause of this serious condition.

Several lines of evidence subsequently established a causal relationship between contrast MRI procedures and the development NSF among patients with advanced kidney disease. Specifically, gadolinium, a component of the contrast media used for MRI procedures, was discovered to be the likely culprit based on several noteworthy findings:

- NSF occurred after only gadolinium MRI procedures.
- Higher amounts of administered gadolinium were associated with greater risks of NSF.
- Gadolinium is eliminated by the kidneys and accumulates in kidney disease.
- Skin biopsies from patients with NSF demonstrated free gadolinium in the dermal layer.
- Gadolinium contrast emerged as the MRI contrast agent of choice during the late 1990s, corresponding with the time trend of initial reports of this condition.

The combination of astute observations, epidemiologic studies, and supportive mechanistic evidence strongly suggested gadolinium contrast as the likely cause of NSF. Based on the totality of these findings, the use of gadolinium was sharply curtailed among people with advanced kidney disease, resulting in a precipitous decline in the incidence of NSF. In this instance, no expensive trials were needed to identify the causal factor and remove it from the susceptible population.

1.1   Inferring Causation from Epidemiologic Studies

Associations relating potential risk factors with disease may or may not indicate causal relationships. For example, scores of observational studies reported an association of higher serum cholesterol levels with the development of myocardial infarction (heart attack). Subsequent mechanistic studies in cell and animal models demonstrated that low-density lipoprotein (LDL), cholesterol promotes the development of atherosclerotic plaques, the primary pathologic lesion in myocardial infarction. Ensuing clinical trials determined that medications designed to lower LDL cholesterol levels concomitantly reduced the risk of myocardial infarction and other cardiovascular disease outcomes. In aggregate, these and other lines of evidence implicated LDL cholesterol as a causal risk factor for coronary heart disease.

In contrast, previous studies reported that estrogen use was associated with lower risks of cardiovascular disease among postmenopausal women. These associations motivated a large-scale clinical trial, in which thousands of postmenopausal women were randomly assigned to receive either estrogen treatment or an inert substance packaged to look like estrogen (placebo). Surprisingly, estrogen treatment in this trial *increased* the risk of cardiovascular disease outcomes, suggesting that the initial observational data did *not* convey the true causal effects of estrogen treatment on these outcomes [3]. One possible explanation for the discrepant findings is that women who used estrogen in the observational studies tended to engage in other healthy behaviors, such as regular exercise and adherence to other prescribed medications, which may have accounted for their lower disease risk. Another possible explanation is that observational studies tended to evaluate women who had used estrogen over a long period of time, potentially missing immediate adverse effects of this treatment.

Separating association from causation in research studies is critically important, because the discovery of causal relationships can promote successful strategies for preventing and treating disease. The discovery of LDL cholesterol as a cause of coronary heart disease led to the development of effective treatments that reduced the development and consequences of this serious condition. The identification of gadolinium contrast as the likely cause of NSF resulted in the removal of this risk factor and prevention of the disease among susceptible individuals.

1.2 Factors Favoring an Inference of Causation

Inferring causal relationships in human research studies is often difficult. Causal inference is hindered by the fact that many common diseases, such as cancer and diabetes, are caused by many risk factors, often acting in combination. Moreover, risk factors for human diseases may require long periods of time to cause illness, such as the impact of secondhand smoke exposure on the risk of cancer. The following criteria can be used as a general guide for assessing whether a potential risk factor is likely to be a cause of disease.

1.2.1 Evidence Arising from Randomized Studies

Studies that randomly assign people to one treatment versus another are generally the most powerful way to demonstrate causal relationships. Random assignment is used to balance the characteristics of treated and untreated individuals to increase the likelihood that these groups differ by only the treatment of interest. Differences in disease outcomes observed in the setting of large randomized trials can be reasonably ascribed to the impact of the treatment itself. Unfortunately, randomized studies are limited to interventions that can be assigned to people in a practical manner, such as drugs or procedures, and tend to be conducted among relatively healthy people under specialized environments that may limit their application.

1.2.2 Strength of Association

Observing a strong association between a potential risk factor and a disease increases the likelihood that the risk factor is a cause of the disease. Strength of association differs from statistical significance. For example, an observational study reported that infants who slept in the prone position were 8.8 times more likely to develop sudden infant death syndrome (SIDS) compared with infants who slept supine: relative risk, 8.8 and p-value, 0.001 [4]. Although the p-value is helpful for excluding chance as a possible explanation for these findings, the size of the observed association, a nearly nine times greater risk of SIDS among infants who slept prone versus supine, is important for inferring a causal relationship. One reason that strong associations tend to indicate causation is that there can only be so much bias and error in well-conducted research studies. Although other characteristics of infants who slept in the prone position may have also influenced the risk of SIDS to some degree, and some errors in classifying SIDS compared with other causes of death may have occurred, it is unlikely that such errors would account for the entirety of such a strong association. There is no consensus rule for defining a "strong" association. For the purposes of this book, associations for which the relative risk is greater than 1.5 or less than $1/1.5 = 0.67$ will be considered "strong."

While strong associations can suggest the presence of causal relationships, weak associations should not be summarily dismissed as noncausal. Many common pitfalls in human research studies tend to dilute observed associations, such as evaluation of risk factors that cause disease in only a fraction of the population under study, the inability to measure potential risk factors at the time they are most strongly related to disease, and inadequate length of follow-up.

1.2.3 Temporal Relationship

The case for a causal relationship between a potential risk factor and disease should include demonstration that the risk factor was present before the development of the disease. Temporality is a necessary, but not sufficient, condition for inferring causation. For example, studies linking gadolinium contrast with NSF included confirmation that the disease was absent at the time of gadolinium administration but developed up to several weeks later.

Example 1.1 A study investigated the risk of secondary bladder associated with cyclophosphamide chemotherapy. Patients in the study had previously received treatment for lymphoma and were initially free of bladder cancer at the time they received this treatment [5]. The study found that the receipt of any cyclophosphamide chemotherapy was associated with a 4.5-times greater incidence of bladder cancer over long-term follow-up.

Demonstration that the risk factor, cyclophosphamide, preceded the development of the disease, bladder cancer, supports the hypothesis of a causal relationship.

In contrast, consider a hypothetical study of a new circulating marker, "DP1," and major depressive disorder. The study finds that serum DP1 levels are three times higher among people who have major depression compared with people who do not have this condition. One explanation for these findings is that elevated levels of DP1 are present before the onset of depression and contribute to its development. Alternatively, it is possible that depression causes metabolic changes that subsequently increase circulating levels of DP1. The ambiguous temporal relationship between serum DP1 levels and depression in this study undermines the inference of causality.

1.2.4 Exposure-Varying Association

The case for causal inference is strengthened by evidence demonstrating that greater amounts of a risk factor are associated with progressively higher risks of the disease. For example, the study of cyclophosphamide chemotherapy found that the receipt of *any* cyclophosphamide was associated with a 4.5-times higher incidence of secondary bladder cancer. The study next demonstrated that higher *cumulative dosages of cyclophosphamide* were associated with progressively greater risks of bladder cancer, shown in Table 1.4.

The concept of dose-response need not be limited to studies of medications. For example, a study reported that upper respiratory infections caused by the organism *Streptococcus* were associated with a greater risk of developing a neuropsychiatric syndrome, including Tourette's disorder, in children [6]. The study next showed that greater *numbers* of streptococcal infections were associated with progressively higher risks of neuropsychiatric disorders, strengthening the case for a causal relationship.

1.2.5 Biological Plausibility

Causal inference relies on scientific knowledge to make sense of observed associations. Associations that have proven biologic plausibility based on experimental and mechanistic data are more likely to represent causal relationships than those not supported by such evidence. The observation that higher LDL cholesterol levels are

Table 1.4 Cyclophosphamide dosage and relative risk of secondary cancer

Cumulative cyclophosphamide dosage (grams)	Relative risk of bladder cancer
None	Reference group
1–20	2.4
20–50	6.0
>50	14.5

associated with myocardial infarction was complemented by parallel mechanistic studies that established biological plausibility: animal studies demonstrating LDL cholesterol deposits (plaques) within the coronary arteries, translational human studies showing enlargement of atherosclerotic plaque size in patients with higher LDL cholesterol levels, and clinical trials establishing that LDL cholesterol-lowering medications reduced the risk of cardiovascular outcomes. Analogously, the observed association of gadolinium contrast with NSF was strongly supported by the results of mechanistic studies, including demonstration of gadolinium deposition in the skin of affected patients. These examples highlight the importance of interdisciplinary research for producing high-quality scientific evidence that can advance public health and clinical care.

References

1. Cowper SE, Robin HS, Steinberg SM, Su LD, Gupta S, LeBoit PE. Scleromyxoedema-like cutaneous diseases in renal-dialysis patients. Lancet. 2000;356(9234):1000–1.
2. Grobner T. Gadolinium–a specific trigger for the development of nephrogenic fibrosing dermopathy and nephrogenic systemic fibrosis? Nephrol Dial Transplant. 2006;21(4):1104–8.
3. Rossouw JE, Anderson GL, Prentice RL, et al. Risks and benefits of estrogen plus progestin in healthy postmenopausal women: principal results from the Women's Health Initiative randomized controlled trial. JAMA. 2002;288(3):321–33.
4. Fleming PJ, Gilbert R, Azaz Y, et al. Interaction between bedding and sleeping position in the sudden infant death syndrome: a population based case-control study. BMJ. 1990;301(6743):85–9.
5. Travis LB, Curtis RE, Glimelius B, et al. Bladder and kidney cancer following cyclophosphamide therapy for non-Hodgkin's lymphoma. J Natl Cancer Inst. 1995;87(7):524–30.
6. Mell LK, Davis RL, Owens D. Association between streptococcal infection and obsessive-compulsive disorder, Tourette's syndrome, and tic disorder. Pediatrics. 2005;116(1):56–60.

Chapter 2
Basic Measures of Disease Frequency

Summary of Learning Points

2.1 Prevalence

   2.1.1 Prevalence describes the amount of disease present in a population at a given time.

   2.1.2 Prevalence data are useful for raising awareness of disease and allocating resources.

   2.1.3 Prevalence data alone are insufficient for establishing temporal relationships.

2.2 Incidence

   2.2.1 Incidence describes the new occurrence of disease over time.

      2.2.1.1 Incidence can be expressed as *incidence proportion* or *incidence rate*.

      2.2.1.2 Incidence rates account for person-time.

      2.2.1.3 Incidence rates are preferable for comparing disease occurrence.

   2.2.2 Incidence data can clarify temporal relationships between risk factors and disease.

2.3 Prevalence is defined as the incidence of disease × duration of disease.

2.4 Measures of disease frequency can be stratified by person, place, and time characteristics to gain insight into the disease process.

Measures of disease frequency quantify the burden and development of disease in populations. Two common measures of disease frequency are *prevalence* and *incidence*.

© Springer Nature Switzerland AG 2019
B. Kestenbaum, *Epidemiology and Biostatistics*,
https://doi.org/10.1007/978-3-319-96644-1_2

2.1 Prevalence

2.1.1 Definition of Prevalence

Prevalence measures the amount of a disease that is present in a population at a given time. Specifically, prevalence is defined as the proportion of people in a population who have a particular disease or condition:

$$\text{Prevalence}\,(\%) = \frac{\text{number of people who have disease}}{\text{number of people in population}} \times 100\%$$

Implicit in this definition is that time is "frozen," such that prevalence provides a snapshot of the amount of disease that is present at a specific point in time (point prevalence) or over some specific period of time (period prevalence).

Example 2.1 A study sought to determine the prevalence of anxiety disorder among high school students. Researchers conducted diagnostic interviews among 1710 students from 2 urban and 3 rural high schools in Central Oregon during 1987–1989 [1]. The study found that 54 of the evaluated students met criteria for anxiety disorder.

What is the prevalence of anxiety disorder among these students?

$$\text{Prevalence}\,(\%) = 54 \,/\, 1710 \times 100\% = 3.2\% \,(\text{during}\,1987-1989)$$

Of note, the term "prevalent" is sometimes used in research studies to describe a previous history of chronic diseases or conditions. For example, the term "prevalent stroke" may be used to describe a past history of stroke, because this condition is presumed to be present indefinitely after diagnosis.

2.1.2 Applications of Prevalence Data

Prevalence data are useful for raising awareness of diseases and guiding resource allocation. For example, the prevalence of type II diabetes in the United States reached approximately 10% in 2010, motivating public health measures to reduce the consumption of high calorie beverages and increasing funding toward the development of new diabetes treatments. Prevalence data can also forewarn of impending complications of a disease. The high prevalence of diabetes in the United States alerted the health community to an expected increase in known complications of the disease, which include eye disease, kidney dysfunction, and peripheral neuropathy.

2.1.3 Limitation of Prevalence Measures

Prevalence data alone are insufficient for establishing a temporal relationship between potential risk factors and disease.

Example 2.2 Vitamin D is synthesized by the skin in response to ultraviolet light. Vitamin D deficiency has been linked with chronic inflammation and may promote the development of autoimmune diseases. In a hypothetical study, researchers compare the prevalence of multiple sclerosis, a chronic relapsing inflammatory disease of the central nervous system, among people who have deficient versus normal levels of vitamin D in a large population.

Prevalence of multiple sclerosis
Vitamin D deficient individuals   0.3%
Vitamin D sufficient individuals   0.1%

At first glance, the relatively higher prevalence of multiple sclerosis among people who are vitamin D-deficient appears to support the possibility of a causal relationship. These prevalence data are compatible with the possibility that vitamin D deficiency occurs before the development of multiple sclerosis, supporting, but not establishing, a causal relationship. However, these same data could also be observed if multiple sclerosis developed first, and then led to a decrease in vitamin D levels, possibly by reducing the amount of time spent outdoors. The prevalence data demonstrate only that vitamin D deficiency and multiple sclerosis tend to be observed together.

2.2 Incidence

2.2.1 Definitions of Incidence

In contrast to prevalence, which provides a static measure of disease burden within a population, incidence describes *new occurrences of disease* over a given period of time. There are two definitions of incidence differing by the choice of denominator:

$$\text{Incidence proportion}\,(\%) = \frac{\text{number of new cases of disease over time}}{\text{population without disease at baseline}} \times 100\%$$

$$\text{Incidence rate}\,(\text{cases per person-time}) = \frac{\text{number of new cases of disease over time}}{\text{person-time at risk}}$$

Incidence proportion is also called *cumulative incidence.*

Example 2.3 Investigators seek to determine the incidence of influenza among nurses at three local hospitals. They identify 500 nurses who do not have influenza as of December 1, 2010, and follow them for the development of influenza over the next 3 months. They find that ten of the study nurses develop influenza during follow-up.

What is the incidence proportion of influenza?

$$\text{Incidence proportion} = \frac{10 \text{ new cases of influenza}}{500 \text{ people initially free of influenza}} \times 100\%$$
$$= 2\% \left(\text{over three} - \text{months} \right)$$

What is the incidence rate of influenza?

Incidence rate has the same numerator as incidence proportion, but the denominator, person-time at risk, requires more in-depth calculation. To demonstrate the calculation of person-time, Fig. 2.1 presents follow-up data for six selected nurses in the study.

Nurses 1 and 3 do not develop influenza over the three month study period. Nurse 2 is followed for 3 months and develops influenza at the end of the study. Nurse 4 develops influenza after only 2 months of follow-up. This person is not considered to be at risk for developing influenza after the disease has occurred in the study (incidence typically counts only one occurrence of disease per person). Nurses 5 and 6 do not develop influenza during the study period but leave the study prematurely, possibly due to relocation or the inability to complete follow-up procedures. These nurses are not considered to be at risk for developing influenza after they drop out, because the study can no longer determine whether or not they develop the disease. Table 2.1 presents person-time data for these six nurses in tabular form.

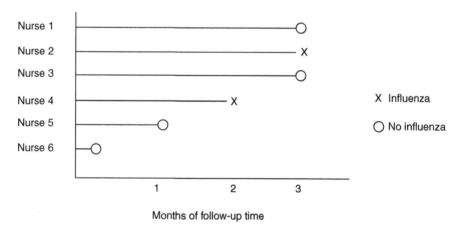

Fig. 2.1 Diagram of individual risk times and disease status

Table 2.1 List of individual risk times and disease status

	Develops influenza	Person-time	Reason for discontinuation
Nurse 1	No	3 months	Study ended
Nurse 2	Yes	3 months	Developed influenza
Nurse 3	No	3 months	Study ended
Nurse 4	Yes	2 months	Developed influenza
Nurse 5	No	1.25 months	Dropped out
Nurse 6	No	0.25 months	Dropped out
Total	2 cases	12.5 months	

For these six individuals:

$$\text{Incidence rate} = \frac{\text{number of new cases of disease}}{\text{person-time at risk}} = \frac{2\,\text{new cases}}{12.5\,\text{months}}$$

$$= 0.16\,\text{cases / month}$$

Incidence rates are typically reported per some rounded measurement of person-time, such as 100 or 1000. The incidence rate of influenza among these six nurses can be multiplied by 100 and reported as 16 cases per 100 person-months.

Calculation of the incidence rate for all 500 nurses in the study requires summation of all the person-time data. Suppose that the total person-time for the 500 nurses in this study is 1200 months. Given a total of 10 new influenza cases that occurred during the study, the incidence rate would be calculated as:

$$\text{Incidence rate} = \frac{\text{number of new cases of disease}}{\text{person-time at risk}} = \frac{10\,\text{new cases}}{1200\,\text{months}}$$

$$= 0.008\,\text{cases / month}$$

Multiplying this incidence rate by 1000 yields a more easily interpretable value of 8 influenza cases per 1000 person-months.

Incidence proportions provide a more interpretable and "user-friendly" description of disease occurrence than incidence rates. On the other hand, incidence rates yield a more precise measurement of disease frequency by accounting for time at risk. For this reason, incidence rates are preferred when *comparing* the occurrence of disease among different groups.

Example 2.4 A study seeks to contrast rates of cellulitis, a common skin infection, among children who are seen at county-based pediatric clinics versus children who are seen at university-based clinics. The researchers identify 500 children who are initially free of cellulitis from each group of clinics and then determine the development of cellulitis over the next 5 years. Results are presented in Table 2.2.

Table 2.2 Comparison of cellulitis incidence in county- and university-based clinics

	Number of children	New cellulitis cases	Person-time
County-based clinics	500	7	1200 years
University-based clinics	500	12	2200 years

Calculation of 5-year incidence proportions reveals a higher incidence of cellulitis among children who are seen at the university clinics.

$$\text{Incidence proportion}\left(\text{county clinics}\right) = \frac{7 \,\text{new cases of cellulitis}}{500 \,\text{without cellulitis at baseline}} \times 100\%$$
$$= 1.4\%$$

$$\text{Incidence proportion}\left(\text{university clinics}\right) = \frac{12 \,\text{new cases of cellulitis}}{500 \,\text{without cellulitis at baseline}} \times 100\%$$
$$= 2.4\%$$

However, these discrepant incidences could have arisen from differences in follow-up time between the groups. Specifically, total person-time was lower in the county clinics, possibly due to higher rates of dropout, relocation, or changes in insurance status. Incidence rates provide a more accurate comparison of the occurrence of cellulitis between the clinics.

$$\text{Incidence rate}\left(\text{county clinic}\right) = \frac{7 \,\text{new cases of cellulitis}}{1200 \,\text{person} - \text{years}}$$
$$= 5.8 \,\text{cases per} \,1000 \,\text{person} - \text{years}$$

$$\text{Incidence rate}\left(\text{university clinic}\right) = \frac{12 \,\text{new cases of cellulitis}}{2200 \,\text{person} - \text{years}}$$
$$= 5.5 \,\text{cases per} \,1000 \,\text{person} - \text{years}$$

The incidence rate of cellulitis is in fact similar among the clinics after accounting for differences in person-time between the groups.

2.2.2 Applications of Incidence Data

By focusing on new occurrences of disease over time, incidence can inform temporal relationships between potential risk factors and disease, supporting inference of causal relationships. For example, consider an alternative approach to the hypothetical study of vitamin D deficiency and multiple sclerosis from Example 2.2.

Example 2.5 A study measures circulating vitamin D levels in a large group of people who are initially free of multiple sclerosis. Over 10 years of follow-up, the incidence rate of multiple sclerosis is found to be 9.3 cases per 10,000 person-years among people who were vitamin D deficient at the start of the study compared with 6.9 cases per 10,000 person-years among people who were vitamin D sufficient.

These contrasting incidence rates support the hypothesis that vitamin D deficiency may contribute to the development of multiple sclerosis, because vitamin D deficiency is present before the onset of the disease. Temporality is but one causal criteria; it remains possible that people who were vitamin D deficient at the beginning of this study possessed other characteristics that predisposed to the higher risk of multiple sclerosis.

2.3   Relationship Between Prevalence and Incidence

The prevalence of a disease within a population at a given time is a function of how frequently the disease occurs (incidence) and how long the disease state lasts (duration). Mathematically,

$$Prevalence = (Incidence) \times (Duration)$$

The relationship between prevalence and incidence is depicted in Fig. 2.2.

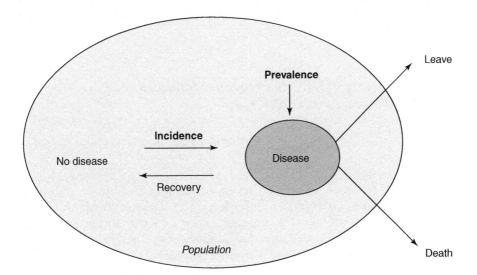

Fig. 2.2 Relationship between prevalence and incidence of disease

Incidence quantifies the *rate* in which people move from the non-diseased to diseased state. Once a person contracts the disease, they may either recover, die from the disease, or leave the population (and can no longer be counted). The prevalence, or burden of disease at a given point in time, is determined by the incidence and the duration of the disease state.

Example 2.6 A hypothetical new treatment is developed for colorectal cancer that arrests tumor growth and dramatically improves survival among patients with the disease. If the incidence of colorectal cancer were to remain constant in the population, what is the expected impact of the new treatment on the prevalence of colorectal cancer?

$$\text{Prevalence} = (\text{Incidence}) \times (\text{Duration})$$

By reducing death due to colorectal cancer, the new treatment would prolong the duration of the disease. Given no change in the incidence of colorectal cancer, the new treatment would be expected to increase the prevalence of this cancer in the population.

2.4   Stratification of Disease Frequencies by Person, Place, and Time

Prevalence and incidence data may be compared across demographics, geographic regions, time periods, or other characteristics to gain insight into a disease process. *Stratification* refers to the process of dividing a population into smaller groups according to specific characteristics.

2.4.1   Measures of Disease Frequency Stratified by Characteristics of Person

Examples of personal characteristics include age, race, and sex. For example, polycythemia vera is a myeloproliferative disorder characterized by an abnormal increase in red blood cell production. The condition is strongly related to age with a prevalence of 163 cases per 100,000 among people aged 75–84 years, compared with only 9 cases per 100,000 among people aged 35–44 years [2]. Moreover, the prevalence of polycythemia vera is greater among men and is particularly high among individuals of Jewish/Eastern European ancestry. These stratified disease frequency measures help define *risk factors* for the disease.

2.4.2 Measures of Disease Frequency Stratified by Characteristics of Place

Variation in disease patterns across geographic regions can also provide clues to the underlying causes of diseases and the responses to treatments. For example, the cumulative incidence of kidney stones is higher in the southeastern United States compared with any other region of the country [3]. Worldwide, the prevalence of kidney stones is inversely related to latitude. This geographic variation is suspected to stem from greater exposure to direct sunlight and heat, which cause dehydration and reduced urine volume that precipitate kidney stone formation.

2.4.3 Measures of Disease Frequency Stratified by Characteristics of Time

Temporal trends in disease rates can also provide clues as to the causes of disease. However, careful consideration must be given to parallel changes in the diagnosis of the condition.

Example 2.7 Cesarean section delivery accounted for approximately 5% of all births in the United States in 1970. By the year 2000, nearly 25% of US babies were born by Cesarean section [4]. One possibility for these temporal changes is an increase in maternal age during this period, leading to more complicated pregnancies requiring Cesarean section. A second possibility is that improved fetal monitoring, which can detect small changes in fetal status, may have prompted more surgical interventions. A third possibility is that routine use of repeat Cesarean section has become standard practice due to data demonstrating a greater risk of uterine rupture for vaginal births performed after a first Cesarean section [5].

Stratified disease frequency measurements are often hypothesis generating in that they motivate further studies to uncover the underlying causes of a condition.

References

1. Lewinsohn PM, Hops H, Roberts RE, Seeley JR, Andrews JA. Adolescent psychopathology: I. Prevalence and incidence of depression and other DSM-III-R disorders in high school students. J Abnorm Psychol. 1993;102(1):133–44.
2. Ania BJ, Suman VJ, Sobell JL, Codd MB, Silverstein MN, Melton LJ 3rd. Trends in the incidence of polycythemia vera among Olmsted County, Minnesota residents, 1935–1989. Am J Hematol. 1994;47(2):89–93.

3. Soucie JM, Thun MJ, Coates RJ, McClellan W, Austin H. Demographic and geographic variability of kidney stones in the United States. Kidney Int. 1994;46(3):893–9.
4. Menacker F. Trends in cesarean rates for first births and repeat cesarean rates for low-risk
   women: United States, 1990–2003. Natl Vital Stat Rep. 2005;54(4):1–8.
5. Lydon-Rochelle M, Holt VL, Easterling TR, Martin DP. Risk of uterine rupture during labor
   among women with a prior cesarean delivery. N Engl J Med. 2001;345(1):3–8.

Chapter 3
General Considerations in Epidemiologic Research

Summary of Learning Points

3.1 Interventional studies assign people to treatments or control procedures, whereas observational studies evaluate exposures that occur naturally.

 3.1.1 Interventional studies can isolate the causal impact of a specific treatment of interest.

 3.1.2 Interventional studies are limited to appraisal of treatments that can be administered to people in a practical and ethical manner.

 3.1.3 Findings obtained from interventional studies may have limited applicability due to the assessment of relatively healthy participants under controlled conditions.

3.2 Study population

 3.2.1 The source population of a research study impacts the applicability of the results.

 3.2.2 Common exclusion criteria include prevalent disease, major risk factors for the disease, inability to obtain valid measurements, and safety.

3.3 Exposure and outcome

 3.3.1 The exposure refers to a characteristic that may explain the outcome of a study.

 3.3.2 The outcome refers to a characteristic that is being predicted in a study.

 3.3.3 Accurate measurements of the study data improve the ability of a study to correctly determine the association of interest.

3.4 Internal and external validity

 3.4.1 Internal validity addresses whether a study accurately answers the proposed question within the specified study population and environment.

 3.4.2 External validity addresses whether the results of a study can be applied to more general groups of people and more inclusive health settings.

© Springer Nature Switzerland AG 2019
B. Kestenbaum, *Epidemiology and Biostatistics*,
https://doi.org/10.1007/978-3-319-96644-1_3

Fundamental considerations in human research studies include the *study design, study population, measurements of the study data, and procedures for follow-up.* These characteristics bear directly on the ability of a study to answer the proposed question of interest.

3.1 Interventional Versus Observational Study Designs

Research study designs can be broadly categorized as interventional versus observational. The distinction arises from the manner in which participants in a study receive treatments or are exposed to potential risk factors. Interventional studies *assign* participants to specific treatments or control procedures typically using a random process. *Randomized trials* are the most common type of interventional study. In contrast, observational studies measure potential risk factors that occur "naturally."

3.1.1 Interventional Studies Can Isolate the Causal Impact of Specific Treatments

The primary advantage of randomized trials is the ability to isolate the *causal effects* of specific treatments by increasing the degree of similarity in participant characteristics across the treatment and control groups.

Example 3.1 Patent foramen ovale (PFO) is a persistent fetal connection between the left and right atria of the heart that fails to close completely after birth. PFO is present in about 25% of the population and is associated with a greater risk of stroke. PFOs can be closed by implanting a specialized device over the defect; however, the impact of PFO closure on stroke prevention is unclear, and the procedure may itself lead to complications, such as an abnormal heart rhythm.

First, consider a hypothetical randomized trial designed to test whether PFO closure reduces the risk of stroke. Such a study could recruit a large number of people with a PFO and then use a random procedure to assign them to either undergo the closure procedure or follow standard medical care. Table 3.1 presents characteristics of participants from a hypothetical randomized trial.

Randomly assigning a large number of people with PFO to either closure or routine care will create similar distributions of characteristics across the intervention groups. Characteristics that might influence a person's decision to undergo PFO closure, such as the size and severity of the PFO or the advice of their physicians, are *not* applicable to whether a participant in this trial is assigned to closure or routine care, because the intervention is assigned at random. Characteristics that are not listed in the table, or even measured in this study, such as dietary habits or health insurance status, are also likely to be similar between participants assigned to

Table 3.1 Baseline characteristics from a hypothetical randomized trial of PFO closure

	Assigned to closure ($N = 1000$)	Assigned to routine care ($N = 1000$)
Age (years)	37.9 ± 15.7	37.5 ± 15.8
Race		
Caucasian	684 (68.4)	691 (69.1)
African American	248 (24.8)	261 (26.1)
Other	68 (6.8)	48 (4.8)
Current smoking	139 (13.9)	144 (14.4)
Family history of diabetes	73 (7.3)	66 (6.6)
Body mass index (kg/m²)	28.9 ± 5.5	28.8 ± 5.5

All values expressed as mean ± standard deviation or number of participants (percent)

Table 3.2 Baseline characteristics from hypothetical observational study of PFO closure

	PFO closure ($N = 520$)	No closure ($N = 1580$)
Age (years)	33.1 ± 19.7	42.7 ± 14.2
Race		
Caucasian	391 (75.3)	1024 (64.8)
African American	87 (16.7)	412 (26.1)
Other	42 (8.0)	144 (9.1)
Current smoking	21 (4.1)	381 (24.1)
Family history of diabetes	37 (7.1)	106 (6.7)
Body mass index (kg/m²)	28.4 ± 6.9	28.9 ± 5.5

closure versus routine medical care due to the random process for assigning these interventions. Assuming that participants who are assigned to PFO closure actually complete this procedure, and those who are assigned to routine care do not, the primary distinction between the groups should be the PFO procedure itself.

Next consider a hypothetical *observational study* to evaluate whether PFO closure is associated with a lower incidence of stroke. Such a study could identify one group of people with a PFO who have undergone the closure procedure and a second group of people with a PFO who have not undergone this procedure. Unlike the interventional study, PFO closure in the observational study is *not* assigned by the researchers, but instead is allowed to occur "naturally," based on the characteristics and preferences of the participants and their caregivers. Table 3.2 presents characteristics from a hypothetical observational study of PFO closure.

The observational study design provides no guarantee that characteristics of people who undergo PFO closure will closely resemble those who do not undergo this procedure. Table 3.2 demonstrates notable differences in age and smoking status between the two groups. Unmeasured characteristics, such as exercise and access to centers that perform the closure procedure, may also differ between these groups. There is no easy way to predict whether unmeasured characteristics will be balanced in an observational study and *increasing the number of participants will have no effect on this uncertainty.*

Table 3.3 Stroke outcomes in the hypothetical randomized interventional study

	Stroke rate (events per 100 person-years)
PFO closure	4.0
Routine care	6.0
	Relative risk = 4.0/6.0 = 0.67

Table 3.4 Stroke outcomes in the hypothetical observational study

	Stroke rate (events per 100 person-years)
PFO closure	2.9
Routine care	8.1
	Relative risk = 2.9/8.1 = 0.36

The degree of similarity among treatment groups bears directly on the interpretation of results obtained from interventional and observational studies. Table 3.3 presents the association of PFO closure with stroke incidence in the hypothetical randomized trial.

The lower incidence of stroke with PFO closure seen in the large randomized trial can be reasonably attributed to the impact of the closure procedure itself on this outcome. There is little concern that the observed difference in stroke incidence could be appreciably distorted by differences in the characteristics of people assigned to closure versus routine care becaue such characteristics are balanced by the randomized study design.

Next, consider the association of PFO closure with stroke seen in the hypothetical observational study, shown in Table 3.4.

Interpretation of the observational data is less certain, because the difference in stroke incidence may be distorted by differences in the characteristics of people who chose to undergo the closure procedure compared with those who did not. The observed association of PFO closure with stroke may or may not indicate a causal impact of this procedure on stroke. Inference for a causal relationship derives from many factors, including the strength of the association, temporality, and biologic plausibility determined from other studies. The above finding would constitute a reasonable starting point in demonstrating a strong and temporal association between PFO closure and a lower incidence of stroke.

3.1.2 Interventional Studies Are Limited to Evaluation of Specific Treatments and Diseases

Randomized trials are useful tools for appraising the risks and benefits of treatments that can be administered to people in a practical and ethical manner. The hypothesis that PFO closure can reduce the incidence of stroke *can* be tested in a randomized trial, because the closure procedure can be feasibly assigned to people in a trial, and because the values and harms of this procedure are uncertain (before conducting the trial), providing ethical justification for assigning participants with a PFO to control procedures (routine care). In contrast, many potential risk factors for human diseases cannot be assigned to people in a practical or ethical manner, such as smoking, high blood pressure, bacterial infections, and inherited genetic sequences. The evaluation of such exposures is limited to observational studies and supportive evidence.

Example 3.2 Metabolic studies provide conflicting data regarding the impact of caffeine intake on the risk of diabetes. On one hand, caffeine can acutely impair glucose tolerance. On the other hand, long-term consumption of caffeinated beverages can increase energy expenditure. Researchers assessed the association of coffee consumption with the incidence of type II diabetes in an observational study of 125,000 health professionals [1]. The study found that greater amounts of coffee consumption were associated with a lower incidence of type II diabetes over 18 years of follow-up.

This study question would be difficult to address using an interventional design, because it would be impractical to assign large numbers of people to different amounts of coffee consumption and enforce this behavior over such a long period of time.

3.1.3 The Results of Interventional Studies May Have Limited Applicability

The causality ascribed to results obtained from large randomized trials may be persuasive for believing that such studies should be used exclusively in research. However, randomized trials are subject to their own limitations, including preferential evaluation of select groups of people within closely monitored environments, relatively short duration of follow-up, and expense. There is near limitless knowledge to be gained from careful observation of the natural variation that exists among people, including genetics, behaviors, medication use, and environmental exposures. In many instances, observational studies are important tools for investigating disease processes and generating novel hypotheses about the prevention and treatment of diseases that can be subsequently tested in interventional studies. Observational studies also have the potential advantage of evaluating potential risk factors and treatments in "real-world" settings, thereby generating results that are broadly applicable to public health.

3.2 Study Population

The term *study population* (also called the *patient population*) refers to *all people who enter a research study*, regardless of whether they are exposed, treated, develop the disease outcome, or drop out after the study begins. The study population originates from a larger *source population*, which is then narrowed using *exclusion criteria*.

3.2.1 Source Population

Participants in research studies may be recruited from a variety of settings, including clinics, hospitals, and communities, depicted in Fig. 3.1. Identifying participants from a single clinic or hospital can provide a convenient and expeditious strategy for recruitment. However, clinical care settings tend to overrepresent people who have more serious diseases and may include specialized practice patterns that may not be applicable to general healthcare settings.

The following examples illustrate how the source population influences the *applicability* of results obtained in research studies to more general groups of people. Applicability is also called *external validity*.

Example 3.3 Clinic-based study of methicillin-resistant *Staphylococcus aureus* in children

Study population	30 consecutive children diagnosed with a staphylococcal soft tissue infection from outpatient pediatric clinics in greater Minneapolis
Study findings	12 of the 30 children (40%) had methicillin-resistant *Staphylococcus aureus*

Clinic-based studies such as this can be relatively easy to conduct, because potential participants are readily accessible to the investigators and relevant data may already be available as part of clinical practice. However, findings from these types of studies may be poorly applicable to other populations. The frequency of methicillin-resistant *Staphylococcus aureus* in this study would be specific to the greater Minneapolis area and influenced by the antibiotic prescription practices of these clinics. The results of this study are likely to apply only to children who live

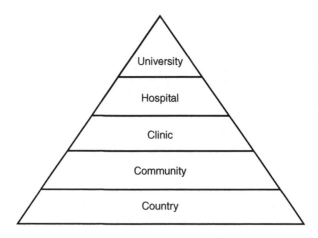

Fig. 3.1 Potential source populations for human research studies

in this geographic area and receive healthcare from clinics with similar practice patterns.

Example 3.4 Health network-based study of hip fracture in chronic kidney disease

Study population   Male veterans receiving care at one of eight Veterans Affairs facilities in Washington State, Idaho, Oregon, and Alaska
Study findings   Late-stage chronic kidney disease is associated with a four times higher incidence of hip fracture.

Health network-based studies such as this offer improved applicability compared with clinic-based studies. In this example, the association between kidney disease and hip fracture is not limited to the practice patterns of a particular clinic, but is more broadly applicable to male veterans who receive regular health care. On the other hand, the study population consists of predominantly older men. Results of the study may not apply to women, who have substantially greater risks of fracture, or to younger people.

Example 3.5 Community-based study of carotid artery disease and cognitive impairment

Study population   Participants from the Cardiovascular Health Study (CHS), a cohort study of 5888 community-living adults aged 65 years and older. The CHS recruited participants from communities across the United States using random sampling from Medicare eligibility lists.
Study findings   High-grade stenosis of the internal carotid arteries is associated with cognitive impairment and cognitive decline over follow-up.

Community-based studies such as this are generally the most complex and expensive to perform, because they involve leaving the healthcare system for the community. The results of such studies tend to have the greatest applicability, because many people in a community never see a doctor, let alone a hospital or university. The observed association of carotid artery disease with cognitive impairment in this study is broadly applicable to older adults in the United States (though possibly not elsewhere), not just those who receive healthcare.

3.2.2 Exclusion Criteria

Following the selection of a source population, research studies typically apply *exclusion criteria* to tailor the study population to the question of interest. General categories of exclusion criteria include prevalent disease, the presence of other risk factors for the disease, the inability to obtain reliable study data, and (in interventional studies) concerns regarding safety.

3.2.2.1 Exclusion of People Who Have Prevalent Disease

Evidence for a causal relationship between a potential risk factor and disease should include demonstration that risk factor was present before the development of the disease (temporal association). This causal criterion is addressed by measuring potential risk factors in people who are free of the disease outcome at the start of a study. For example, the study of coffee consumption and type II diabetes excluded people who initially had a diagnosis of diabetes, when levels of coffee consumption were measured. This exclusion increases the degree of certainty that coffee consumption habits preceded the occurrence of diabetes in the study.

3.2.2.2 Exclusion of People Who Have Another Strong
Risk Factor for the Disease

In some instances, the case for a causal relationship between a risk factor and disease can be strengthened by excluding people who have other strong risk factors for the disease. For example, the observed association of coffee consumption with a lower incidence of type II diabetes is subject to distortion by the presence of obesity, which could be related to the amount of coffee consumption, and is a strong risk factor for diabetes. The researchers could minimize the potential distorting influence of this risk factor by excluding people with obesity.

Exclusion for other disease risk factors enhances the ability of a study to focus on a specific risk factor of interest but can diminish the applicability of the study results. Excluding people who have obesity from the coffee consumption study would generate results that apply exclusively to nonobese individuals, lessening the health impact of the findings. It is also possible that coffee consumption has particularly important effects on diabetes among people who are obese; this possibility would be missed by exclusion. In practice, exclusion for disease risk factors represents a carefully judged balance between internal validity, the ability of a study to reliably answer the proposed question of interest, including the ability to measure and adjust for other causal factors, and external validity, the ability of a study to generate findings that are broadly applicable to more general groups of people and healthcare settings.

3.2.2.3 Exclusion of People Who Cannot Provide Reliable Study Data

It is usually necessary to limit the study population to people who can provide reliable data needed to conduct the study. For example, the study of coffee consumption obtained information regarding this exposure from mailed questionnaires that inquired about the typical number of cups of coffee consumed per day. People who did not return these questionnaires, and people who reported implausible information, were excluded. Analogously, randomized trials often exclude people who are expected to have difficulties completing the planned study procedures, such as people with extensive comorbidities or major physical or cognitive disabilities.

3.2.2.4   Exclusion of People Who Cannot Complete the Study Safely

Clinical trials that administer tests, procedures, or treatments must necessarily exclude people who cannot safely complete these interventions. For example, a study to evaluate the impact of a new dementia treatment on white matter changes within the brain, as determined by magnetic resonance imaging (MRI), would exclude people who cannot safely undergo the MRI procedure due to specific metallic implants or claustrophobia.

3.2.3   *Where to Find Information About the Study Population in a Research Article*

Details of the study population are typically presented in the first paragraphs of the methods section of a research article. Ideally, this section should define the underlying source population and detail the specific exclusion criteria. Research articles may also use a flowchart to present the study population and exclusions, shown in Fig. 3.2 for the coffee consumption study.

This information is often useful for appraising the external validity of the study findings. A large number of excluded people relative to the number initially evaluated can suggest caution in applying the results of the study to more general populations with the condition of interest.

3.3   Exposure and Outcome

3.3.1   *Definition*

The terms *exposure* and *outcome* are commonly applied to studies of disease causation, treatment, and prognosis. The *exposure* of a study refers to *any characteristic that may explain or predict the presence of a study outcome*. Examples of exposures include blood pressure, smoking, viral infections, and serum cholesterol levels. In observational studies, exposures may also be called "risk factors." The *outcome* of a study refers to the characteristic that is being predicted. The study outcome is often a disease but can be any characteristic, such as the change in tumor size, severity of depression symptoms, or survival. The distinction between

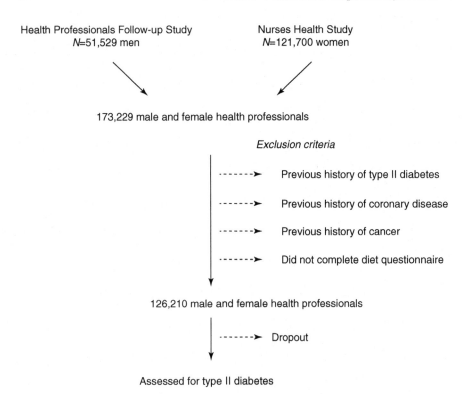

Fig. 3.2 Flow chart of study population from study of coffee consumption and diabetes

exposure and outcome depends on the study question, as demonstrated by the following examples.

Example 3.6 An observational study examines the effectiveness of a vaccine designed to prevent streptococcal pneumonia. Researchers review the medical records of 1500 patients to determine whether or not they received the vaccine and whether they developed streptococcal pneumonia during follow-up. The study question is:

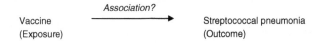

The exposure in this study is the receipt of the vaccine (yes *versus* no) and the outcome is the development of streptococcal pneumonia.

Example 3.7 An observational study investigates whether household income is associated with the regular use of herbal medications. Investigators recruit 500 people from a local shopping mall and administer questionnaires that inquire about household income and patterns of herbal medication use. The study question is:

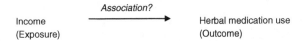

Note that the outcome being predicted in this study is the use of a medication. Other studies may evaluate medication use as the exposure to determine associations with disease.

Example 3.8 A clinical trial tests whether the placement of a coronary stent, a device used to enhance blood flow to the heart, improves survival following a myocardial infarction (heart attack). The investigators use a random procedure to assign 1000 patients who experienced a first myocardial infarction to either receive a coronary stent or follow routine cardiac care. Study participants are followed over time to assess survival. The study question is:

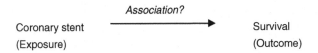

In the context of this clinical trial, the exposure, coronary stent placement, would be called the *study treatment* or *study intervention*. The outcome of this study is survival.

3.3.2 Measuring the Study Data

In most human research studies, idealized measurements of the study data, including the exposure, outcome, and other information relevant to the study, may be difficult to obtain. For example, the study of coffee consumption and type II diabetes estimated the amount of coffee intake using mailed questionnaires that inquired about the average amount of coffee consumed in a typical day. Coffee consumption reported on these questionnaires may differ from the actual coffee consumption habits of the participants. Similar considerations apply to the outcome of the study, type II diabetes, which was ascertained by participant self-report.

Errors in measuring the study data can undermine the ability of a study to correctly determine the association of interest. Typically, errors in measuring the exposure or the outcome of a study will produce the largest distortions in the observed association, and larger errors in these measurements will tend to produce more bias. The specific impact of measurement error on the results of studies is discussed in Chap. 9.

Accuracy describes the degree to which a measured characteristic reflects the *true value* of that characteristic. Accuracy can be assessed by comparing the results of study measurements to the findings obtained from a *gold-standard* method. Gold-standard procedures are often invasive, expensive, and impractical to apply to large populations but can be performed in smaller groups of people to assess the accuracy of more realistic measurements. For example, a gold-standard procedure to determine the occurrence of type II diabetes is review of medical records to identify diagnostic criteria for this condition, including an elevated fasting glucose level, an abnormal response to a glucose tolerance test, or the initiation of a medication to treat diabetes. Researchers in the coffee consumption study obtained medical records from a small sample of participants who reported developing diabetes during the study. They found confirmatory diagnostic evidence for type II diabetes in 98%. The researchers also invited a small number of participants who did not report the occurrence of diabetes to undergo glucose tolerance testing. Less than 1% were found to have undiagnosed diabetes. These results provide justification for the use of self-report to determine the occurrence of type II diabetes in the full study population.

There is no gold-standard method for measuring the amount of coffee consumption over a long period of time. Nonetheless, the quality of the data obtained from the mailed questionnaires can be indirectly appraised by comparison with the results of more detailed measurements. Researchers in the study asked a small group of participants to maintain prospective diaries of all foods and beverages consumed over 1 week. They found excellent agreement between coffee consumption recorded in these diaries and coffee consumption reported in the mailed questionnaires in participants who completed both procedures.

3.3.3   Where to Find Information About the Exposure and Outcome in a Research Article

Details regarding the exposure and outcome of a study, and the procedures used to measure these characteristics, are typically found in the methods section of a research article (following the description of the patient population). This section should describe how the study data were collected and report the accuracy of the measurements, if such information is known.

3.4   Internal and External Validity

Internal validity addresses the degree to which a study correctly answers the proposed question within the given population and environment. A simple way to think of internal validity is to ask, "are the results of the study likely to be *true*?" Examples of strategies used to increase internal validity include the use of a randomized design to isolate the causal impact of a specific treatment (if applicable), exclusions for major disease risk factors, procedures to encourage adherence with the study treatments, appropriate statistical analyses, and detailed methods to measure the exposure, outcome, and other study data with a high degree of certainty.

External validity, also called *applicability* or *generalizability*, addresses whether the results of a study are likely to be broadly applicable to more general groups of people and more realistic environments. A simple way to think of external validity is to ask, "can I apply the results of this study to other health settings or to the patients I see in my practice?" Strategies used to increase the external validity of studies include community-based recruitment, broad inclusion criteria with few exclusions, and practical monitoring strategies that can be readily duplicated in real-world settings. The results from externally valid studies have the greatest potential to impact healthcare.

Some characteristics may have opposing influences on internal and external validity. Consider the hypothetical randomized trial comparing PFO closure to routine care from Example 3.1. Researchers conducting the trial could frequently contact participants assigned to routine medical care to encourage adherence with standard therapies for stroke prevention, including blood pressure control and the regular use of aspirin. Procedures to promote compliance could increase the internal validity of the trial by increasing the likelihood that the participants truly received their assigned treatments. On the other hand, consistent reminders to encourage adherence are *not* representative of real-world medical care. It is possible that such procedures could lead to a lower incidence of stroke among people assigned to routine medical care in the randomized trial compared with those who receive routine care in more realistic settings. Consequently, the relative benefit of PFO closure on stroke reduction observed in the trial might be smaller than the real-world impact of this procedure, reducing the external validity of the trial findings.

Analogously, exclusion for major disease risk factors can increase the internal validity of a study while reducing external validity. In the hypothetical observational study of PFO closure and stroke, the researchers might consider performing carotid ultrasounds to measure the amount of atherosclerosis, a strong risk factor for stroke, at the start of study, and then excluding people who are found to have this risk factor. Exclusion for carotid artery disease would increase the internal validity of the study by enhancing focus on the impact of the PFO closure procedure itself on stroke. However, excluding people with carotid artery disease would diminish the external validity of the results, because they would not apply to the many people who have a PFO and coexisting carotid artery disease.

3.5 Summary of Common Research Study Designs

Figure 3.3 provides an overview of the common research study designs covered in this book. Details of these specific designs, along with their inherent strengths and weaknesses, are described in subsequent chapters.

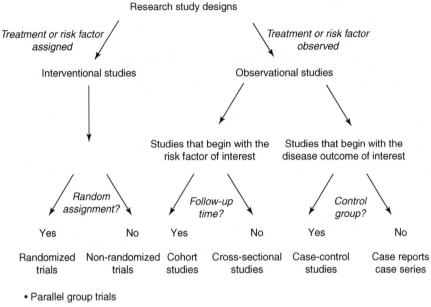

Fig. 3.3 General overview of common research study designs

Reference

1. Salazar-Martinez E, Willett WC, Ascherio A, et al. Coffee consumption and risk for type 2 diabetes mellitus. Ann Intern Med. 2004;140(1):1–8.

Chapter 4
Case Reports and Case Series

Summary of Learning Points

4.1 Case reports and case series are observational studies that describe the experience of one or more people with a particular disease or condition.

4.2 Case reports and case series can be an important first step in recognizing a new disease.

4.3 Case reports and case series have specific limitations:

    4.3.1 Lack of denominator data needed to calculate disease incidence

    4.3.2 Lack of a comparison group

    4.3.3 Select study populations

    4.3.4 Sampling variation

Case reports and case series represent the most basic types of observational study designs. These studies describe the experiences of a single person (*case report*) or a group of people (*case series*) who have a specific disease or condition. Case reports and case series typically describe previously unrecognized diseases or unusual variants of a known disease process. Consequently, data from these studies are particularly useful for alerting the health community to the presence of a new disease and for generating hypotheses regarding possible causes. For example, initial case reports of opportunistic infections among previously healthy homosexual men alerted the health community to the presence of the human immunodeficiency virus (HIV) epidemic. The initial case series describing patients with nephrogenic systemic fibrosis (NSF) raised awareness of this previously unknown condition and motivated subsequent studies that ultimately led to the discovery of gadolinium contrast as the causal agent (Chap. 1).

Case reports and case series can provide compelling reading, because they often present detailed accounts of the experiences of individual people. However, these studies have inherent limitations that reduce their utility to discern causal relationships.

© Springer Nature Switzerland AG 2019
B. Kestenbaum, *Epidemiology and Biostatistics*,
https://doi.org/10.1007/978-3-319-96644-1_4

Example 4.1 A case series described 15 women who developed an aggressive form of breast cancer. Nine of these women reported the recent ingestion of foods packaged with the chemical bisphenol A (BPA). This substance exhibits carcinogenic and estrogenic properties in animal models. Urine testing confirmed the presence of BPA in all nine of these women.

The results of this case series are important for raising awareness of BPA as a possible new risk factor for breast cancer. However, the study data are insufficient for inferring a causal relationship between BPA exposure and cancer.

First, case reports and case series *lack denominator data* needed to calculate the incidence of disease. Recall that incidence is defined as the number of new cases of a disease divided by the number of people who are initially free of the disease (incidence proportion) or person-time (incidence rate). The incidence proportion of breast cancer among women who are exposed to BPA would be defined as:

$$\text{Incidence proportion}(\%) = \frac{\text{number of new breast cancers in women exposed to BPA}}{\text{total number of women exposed to BPA}} \times 100\%$$

The case series data include the numerator: nine new cases of breast cancer among women who were exposed to BPA but provide no information regarding the denominator, the total number of women exposed to BPA from whom these breast cancer cases arose. The inability to determine the incidence of disease precludes valid comparison of breast cancer occurrence between women who are exposed to BPA and those who are not exposed. Obtaining necessary denominator information may not be easy. In this example, additional data sources would be needed to determine the total number of BPA exposed women from whom these cancer cases developed.

A second problem with case report and case series data is the lack of a comparison group. Among the 15 women with breast cancer in the case series, 9 (60%) were found to have been exposed to BPA. This frequency appears to be high; however, BPA is a newly recognized chemical that is commonly used in many types of food packaging. Knowledge of the frequency of BPA exposure among women who do *not* develop breast cancer would be necessary to determine an association.

A third limitation of case reports and case series is the tendency to describe disease processes among unique individuals who may not represent "typical" people with the same disease. For example, the women with breast cancer in the case series may have been selected from a single university hospital that provides referral care for refractory or highly aggressive cancers. The 60% frequency of BPA exposure among these women may reflect specific characteristics of patients who are treated at this particular hospital.

A fourth limitation of case reports and case series is *sampling variation*. The 15 women with breast cancer in this case series are but a small sample of all similar women who have breast cancer from the larger underlying population. Selecting different random samples of 15 women from this larger population will result in variable proportions of BPA exposure due to chance alone. More precise estimates of disease and exposure frequencies, independent from chance, require greater numbers of study subjects.

Recall the criteria used to judge causal inference:

- Evidence arising from randomized studies
- Strong association between potential risk factor and disease
- Temporal relationship
- Exposure or dose varying association
- Biological plausibility

Case reports and case series rely on biologic plausibility from other studies and, in some instances, temporal relationships to make the case for causation. For the case series of BPA exposure and breast cancer, there is no randomized evidence, no measure of association between BPA exposure and cancer, no indication that exposure to BPA preceded the development of cancer, and no data regarding a possible dose-response. Presumption of a causal relationship in this instance derives completely from prior biologic knowledge regarding the potential estrogenic and carcinogenic effects of BPA.

Despite their limitations, case reports and case series may be highly suggestive of new associations, disease processes, or unintended side effects of medications or treatments.

Example 4.2 In 2007, a case series described male prepubertal gynecomastia (an increase in the size of male breast tissue) among three otherwise healthy boys [1]. All were found to have recently used products containing lavender oil. The condition resolved after discontinuation of the lavender oil product in all cases. Previous experimental studies suggested that lavender oil mimics properties of estrogen, a hormone that promotes breast tissue growth.

Limitations of case series data apply to the results of this study: the number of cases is small, and no data is provided regarding the frequency of lavender oil exposure among boys who do not develop gynecomastia. Nonetheless, support for a possible causal role of lavender oil in the development of gynecomastia derives not only from biologic plausibility but also from demonstration of a temporal relationship between this exposure and the disease process. The boys in this case series were previously healthy prior to the use of lavender oil, and the condition resolved after discontinuation of this exposure. These initial case series data prompted further studies of lavender oil, a common ingredient in commercially available products such as soaps and shampoos, as a potential cause of gynecomastia.

Example 4.3 Following commercial release of a vaccine designed to prevent rotavirus infection, several cases of intussusception, a rare condition in which one portion of the bowel slides into the next, were reported among young children soon after vaccination [2]. In preclinical testing, the vaccine was found to cause weakening of the intestinal muscle layers in animal models.

Intussusception is typically a rare condition. The temporal occurrence of this disease following a particular exposure combined with highly suggestive experimental evidence provides a strong case for a causal relationship. The strong biologic plausibility underlying this association, knowledge that intussusception is an otherwise rare condition, and demonstration of a temporal relationship between receipt of the vaccine and intussusception were highly suggestive of a causal impact of the vaccine on this outcome. Based on these and other similar findings, the vaccine was subsequently removed from the market.

References

1. Henley DV, Lipson N, Korach KS, Bloch CA. Prepubertal gynecomastia linked to lavender and tea tree oils. N Engl J Med. 2007;356(5):479–85.
2. Centers for Disease C, Prevention. Intussusception among recipients of rotavirus vaccine–United States, 1998–1999. MMWR Morb Mortal Wkly Rep. 1999;48(27):577–81.

Chapter 5
Cross-Sectional Studies

Summary of Learning Points
5.1 Cross-sectional studies are observational studies in which the exposure and outcome are measured at the same time.
5.2 Cross-sectional studies can determine associations of exposures with disease prevalence.
5.3 Cross-sectional studies cannot establish a temporal relationship between the exposure and outcome of a study, unless one direction of association is implausible.

Cross-sectional studies are a type of observational study in which the exposure and outcome are measured simultaneously. Contemporaneous measurement of potential risk factors and a disease outcome implies that there is *no follow-up time in cross-sectional studies.*

Example 5.1 Homocysteine, an amino acid formed during conversion of methionine to cysteine, exhibits pro-inflammatory and pro-thrombotic properties. A study evaluated the association of circulating homocysteine levels with peripheral arterial disease in 6744 men and women from a large primary care network in Germany [1]. The researchers quantified serum homocysteine levels using high-performance liquid chromatography and assessed the presence of peripheral arterial disease by measuring blood pressures in the ankles and arms. An ankle-to-arm blood pressure ratio less than 0.9 was considered to represent evidence of peripheral arterial disease. The results of the study are presented in Table 5.1.

The investigators divided measured homocysteine levels into *quintiles* or five groups of roughly equal size. The data in Table 5.1 describe the amount of peripheral arterial disease that is present among people in each homocysteine category at the time these levels were measured. Recall that prevalence describes the amount of

© Springer Nature Switzerland AG 2019
B. Kestenbaum, *Epidemiology and Biostatistics*,
https://doi.org/10.1007/978-3-319-96644-1_5

Table 5.1 Association of serum homocysteine levels with peripheral arterial disease

Serum homocysteine level (umol/L)	Peripheral arterial disease		Total
	Present	Absent	
<10.6	177	1176	1353
10.6–13.0	224	1123	1347
13.0–15.5	228	1122	1350
15.5–19.1	259	1090	1349
>19.1	325	1020	1345

disease that is present in a population at a specific time. The prevalence of peripheral arterial disease among participants in the highest serum homocysteine category can be calculated as:

$$\text{Prevalence}\,(\%) = \frac{\text{number of people who have disease}^*}{\text{number of people in population}}\,100\%$$

$$= \frac{325}{(1020 + 325)}\,100\% = 24.2\%$$

Analogously, the prevalence of peripheral arterial disease among participants in the lowest serum homocysteine category can be calculated as:

$$\text{Prevalence}\,(\%) = \frac{\text{number of people who have disease}^*}{\text{number of people in population}}\,100\%$$

$$= \frac{177}{(1176 + 177)}\,100\% = 13.1\%$$

On the other hand, cross-sectional study data *cannot* be used to calculate incidence, which describes the occurrence of new disease over time, because there is no follow-up time in cross-sectional studies.

The cross-sectional data in Table 5.1 can be used to compare the prevalence of peripheral arterial disease among different categories of serum homocysteine levels.

$$\text{Prevalence ratio} = \frac{\text{Prevalence in exposed population}}{\text{Prevalence in unexposed population}}$$

For example, the prevalence of peripheral arterial disease comparing participants in the highest versus lowest quintile of serum homocysteine levels would be calculated as:

$$\text{Prevalence ratio} = \frac{\text{Prevalence in exposed population}}{\text{Prevalence in unexposed population}}\frac{24.2\%}{13.1\%} = 1.8\,(\text{no units})$$

The choice of exposed and unexposed populations is flexible and depends on the study question. For the purposes of this example, participants who had the highest serum homocysteine levels were selected as the exposed population to convey the greater risk of disease associated with this exposure. The prevalence ratio can be interpreted as, "the highest quintile of serum homocysteine levels is associated with a 1.8-times greater prevalence of peripheral arterial disease compared with the lowest quintile."

This observed association may or may not represent a causal impact of homocysteine levels on the development of peripheral arterial disease. Recall the criteria used to judge causal inference:

- Evidence arising from randomized studies
- Strong association between potential risk factor and disease
- Temporal relationship
- Exposure or dose varying association
- Biological plausibility

The homocysteine and peripheral arterial disease study is not randomized; it is not possible to assign people to specific circulating homocysteine levels (though it may be possible to assign people to treatments that lower homocysteine levels). The observed association, comparing the highest to lowest homocysteine categories, is reasonably "strong," based on a prevalence ratio >1.5. Moreover, the data in Table 5.1 demonstrate a consistently higher prevalence of peripheral arterial disease associated with successively greater serum homocysteine levels, providing evidence of an exposure-varying association. Biological plausibility for the association is supported by data from previous mechanistic studies, which demonstrate pro-inflammatory and pro-thrombotic effects of homocysteine that may contribute to atherosclerosis.

What about a temporal relationship? Ideally, evidence to support a causal role of homocysteine in the development of peripheral arterial disease would include demonstration that this exposure was present before the occurrence of the disease. The cross-sectional data are compatible with the possibility that higher serum homocysteine levels precede the development of peripheral arterial disease. However, these data are also compatible with the possibility that peripheral arterial disease occurs first and then promotes secondary metabolic responses that include an increase in homocysteine levels. There is no way to distinguish between these possibilities from the cross-sectional data alone, depicted in Fig. 5.1.

The concept that the outcome of a study may itself influence the exposure is called *reverse causality*. This limitation is inherent to the cross-sectional study

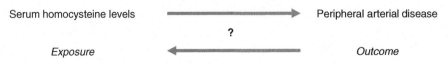

Fig. 5.1 Ambiguous direction of association in a cross-sectional study

Table 5.2 Association of sex with peripheral arterial disease

	Peripheral arterial disease	
	Present	Absent
Women	655	3243
Men	564	2282

design, due to simultaneous measurement of the exposure and outcome, and cannot be overcome by any statistical method of correction. Nonetheless, the possibility of reverse causality may be of little concern in some cross-sectional studies if one direction of causality is implausible. For example, consider a study that compares the prevalence of peripheral arterial disease in men versus women (Table 5.2).

$$\text{Prevalence of peripheral arterial disease in women} = 655/(655+3243)*100\%$$
$$= 16.8\%$$

$$\text{Prevalence of peripheral arterial disease in men} = 564/(564+2282)*100\%$$
$$= 19.8\%$$

$$\text{Prevalence ratio} = 16.8\% / 19.8\% = 0.85$$

Women in this study have a 15% lower prevalence of peripheral arterial disease compared with men. In this instance, there is *no* ambiguity regarding a temporal relationship between the exposure and the outcome. It is certain that a person's sex precedes their development of peripheral arterial disease. The alternative possibility that peripheral arterial disease influences whether a person is male or female is biologically implausible. Other examples of characteristics that clearly precede the development of disease and can be readily assessed as exposures in cross-sectional studies include inherited genetic sequences, race, and age.

Despite the inherent inability of many cross-sectional studies to discern temporal relationships, this design remains popular because it can utilize existing data from more laborious study designs and often obtains results immediately, without waiting for the accrual of follow-up data.

Example 5.2 Researchers conducted a clinical trial to test whether dietary fiber supplementation can reduce the risk of colorectal cancer. They identified eligible persons who were initially free of cancer, randomly assigned them to receive either dietary fiber supplements or no such treatment, and then compared the incidence of new colorectal cancers over 10 years of follow-up.

The researchers could perform additional analyses related to colorectal cancer while waiting for accrual of the long-term outcome data. For example, stool samples collected at the start of the trial could be used to detect the presence of specific colonic microorganisms and these findings assessed for associations with serum levels of carcinoembryonic antigen (CEA), a marker of early colorectal cancer. Such a hypothetical cross-sectional study would be unable to clarify whether the identified microorganisms preceded the levels of CEA or vice versa. However, the study would be immediately feasible and could generate new hypotheses regarding potential anticancer mechanisms of dietary fiber.

Reference

1. Darius H, Pittrow D, Haberl R, et al. Are elevated homocysteine plasma levels related to peripheral arterial disease? Results from a cross-sectional study of 6880 primary care patients. Eur J Clin Investig. 2003;33(9):751–7.

Chapter 6
Cohort Studies

Summary of Learning Points

6.1 Cohort studies are observational studies that are conducted in three fundamental steps:

    6.1.1 Exclude people who have the disease outcome at the start of the study

    6.1.2 Measure one or more exposures to define the cohorts

    6.1.3 Determine the incidence of the disease outcome over time

6.2 Ideal measurements of the exposure should be accurate, precise, equitable, and timely.

6.3 Pharmacoepidemiology studies are observational studies that evaluate the consequences of medications or procedures.

6.4 Analysis of cohort study data

    6.4.1 Relative risk is a ratio of disease incidences that describes risk to an individual.

    6.4.2 Attributable risk and population attributable risk are differences in disease incidences that describe risk to a population.

6.5 Advantages of cohort studies include:

    6.5.1 Can discern temporal relationships between exposures and disease

    6.5.2 Can be used to efficiently study multiple disease outcomes

6.6 Limitations of cohort studies include:

    6.6.1 Confounding characteristics other than the exposure of interest may bias observed associations with disease

    6.6.2 Inefficient design for studying rare diseases or those with long latency periods

© Springer Nature Switzerland AG 2019
B. Kestenbaum, *Epidemiology and Biostatistics*,
https://doi.org/10.1007/978-3-319-96644-1_6

6.1   Cohort Study Design

Cohort studies are observational studies that compare the *incidence of disease* among different exposure groups. The cohort study design separates potential risk factors from the development of disease over time to demonstrate temporal associations.

Cohort studies are conducted in three fundamental steps:

1. Identify a group of people who are initially free of the disease outcome
2. Measure the exposure(s) of interest to create cohorts
3. Follow the cohorts over time to determine the incidences of disease

6.1.1   Exclusion for Prevalent Disease

Cohort studies begin by excluding people who have the disease outcome at the beginning of the study. Exclusion for preexisting or *prevalent* disease is intended to support a temporal relationship between the exposure(s) and disease, a condition necessary, though not sufficient, for inferring causal relationships. Consider an alternative approach to the study of serum homocysteine levels and peripheral arterial disease from the previous chapter (Example 5.1).

Example 6.1   Researchers identify 7000 men and women from a multi-site primary care network. They first exclude people who are found to have a previous history of peripheral arterial disease at the start of the study. Next, they measure serum homocysteine levels in the presumably disease-free participants and conduct annual follow-up examinations to ascertain new occurrences of peripheral arterial disease over time.

Measuring serum homocysteine levels in a population that is initially free of peripheral arterial disease increases the likelihood that this exposure is present before the occurrence of the disease. Under the cohort study design, it is unlikely that serum homocysteine levels could be influenced by peripheral arterial disease outcomes, depicted in Fig. 6.1.

In practice, exclusion for prevalent disease may not be easy and increases the complexity of a study. Methods to ascertain the presence of peripheral arterial disease include participant self-report, review of medical record data, and comparison of blood pressures in the ankles and arms. For example, study participants could

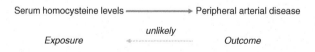

Fig. 6.1   Clear direction of association in a cohort study

complete questionnaires inquiring about previous medical diagnoses, surgeries, and symptoms of peripheral arterial disease, such as pain in the legs with exertion. Alternatively, a history of peripheral arterial disease could be ascertained via medical chart review, if such data were uniformly available for all study participants. The measurement of blood pressures in the ankles and arms can also be used to identify peripheral arterial disease but may be impractical to perform in large studies.

In some instances, cohort studies may strengthen evidence for a temporal association by further excluding people who have *subclinical disease*, which describes early, clinically silent stages of a disease process.

Example 6.2 The kidneys play a central role in regulating blood pressure. A cohort study evaluated the association of kidney function with the development of hypertension among adults from six US communities [1]. The investigators first excluded people who had prevalent hypertension at the start of the study, defined by a systolic blood pressure≥140 mmHg, a diastolic blood pressure ≥90 mmHg, or the use of a medication for hypertension. To increase the degree of certainty that the exposure, kidney function, was measured before the onset of hypertension, the investigators further excluded people who had subclinical or "borderline" hypertension, defined by a systolic blood pressure 120–140 mmHg or a diastolic pressure 80–90 mmHg (note that definitions of hypertension have since changed). The study found that lower kidney function at the start of the study was associated with a greater probability of developing hypertension over follow-up.

6.1.2 Creation of the Cohorts

As a type of observational study, cohort studies ascertain exposures that occur "naturally." Measurement of the exposure of interest classifies participants into *cohorts*, which are defined as groups of people derived from the study population who share a common experience or condition and whose outcomes are unknown at the start of the study.

Example 6.3 A fictitious new antibiotic, "supramycin," is approved for treating pneumonia. A cohort study evaluates whether the use of this antibiotic is associated with the development of a rash. Study investigators review electronic pharmacy records to identify 100 patients with pneumonia who are treated with supramycin and a comparison group of 400 patients with pneumonia who are treated with amoxicillin, an older antibiotic. The investigators follow these cohorts over 4 weeks to ascertain the development of new rashes.

The exposure in this study, antibiotic type (supramycin versus amoxicillin), is determined by review of pharmacy records. Ascertainment of the exposure divides the study population into two mutually exclusive cohorts of supramycin users and amoxicillin users, who are followed prospectively for the occurrence of the outcome, rash, illustrated in Fig. 6.2.

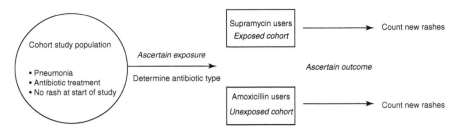

Fig. 6.2 Creation of the cohorts in study of antibiotic type

By convention, cohorts are designated as "exposed" or "unexposed." The definition is flexible and depends on the study question. In this example, supramycin users are designated as the exposed cohort, because this antibiotic is hypothesized to be associated with a higher risk of rash. The number of cohorts need not be limited to two. For example, measurement of serum homocysteine levels in the peripheral arterial disease study (Example 6.1) divides the population into many cohorts, based on the measured value of homocysteine. Continuous exposures such as homocysteine levels, which can take on a theoretically infinite number of values, can be divided into categories, such as those shown in Table 5.1. Exposure categories are often based on accepted definitions, for example, body mass index categories of "normal" (<25 kg/m^2), "overweight" (25–30 kg/m^2), or "obese" (>30 kg/m^2). In the absence of established categories, continuous exposures can be divided into equally sized groups, such as tertiles (three equal groups) or quartiles (four equal groups).

6.1.3   Determination of the Outcome

Cohort studies require follow-up procedures to ascertain outcomes, such as scheduled study examinations, telephone contacts, monitoring of electronic medical records, or linkage with registries. Because cohort studies require the accrual of outcome data over time, these types of studies are typically more complex and laborious to conduct than cross-sectional studies.

Example 6.4 The Multi-Ethnic Study of Atherosclerosis is a prospective cohort study of cardiovascular disease among 6814 community-living adults [2]. All participants were free of clinically apparent cardiovascular disease at the start of the study. The study collected a wealth of exposure data, including measurements of lipids, inflammation, calcification, and cardiac structure. Researchers monitored participants for the development of new cardiovascular events throughout the study via 6-month telephone contacts and annual follow-up examinations. Potential events prompted the collection of hospitalization records, which were reviewed by physicians blinded to the other study data.

Example 6.5 A cohort study evaluated the association of dietary fish consumption with pancreatic cancer [3]. The investigators used food frequency questionnaires to determine the type, amount, and frequency of fish intake in 66,616 adults at the start of the study. Participants were followed prospectively for the development of new pancreatic cancers by linking study records with the Surveillance, Epidemiology, and End Results (SEER) cancer registry, which obtains cancer data from hospitals, oncologists, pathologists, and radiotherapists.

6.2   Quality of the Exposure Measurements

Idealized measurements of study exposures are often impractical or prohibitively expensive to obtain. For example, the study of dietary fish consumption measured this exposure using food frequency questionnaires, which are relative easy to administer but may not perfectly characterize the actual fish consumption habits of the participants. Other methods to determine fish intake, such as the prospective recording of all foods consumed over 1 week with subsequent software analyses or the measurement of fatty acid levels specific to fish intake, may quantify fish consumption more correctly but would be difficult to perform in such a large study. Important considerations for evaluating the quality of exposure measurements include accuracy, precision, equity, and timing.

6.2.1   Are the Measurements Accurate?

Accuracy, or validity, refers to how well a measured characteristic reflects the *true value* of that characteristic. For example, the accuracy of fish intake determined by the food frequency questionnaires refers to how closely these data reflect actual fish consumption. The accuracy of serum homocysteine levels in the peripheral arterial disease study refers to how well these measured levels relate to actual circulating homocysteine levels in the body. Characteristics that could impact the accuracy of the homocysteine measurements include procedures used to collect and store the blood samples and details of the specific laboratory assay. Accuracy can be assessed by comparing the measured values of a characteristic to values obtained from a *gold-standard procedure*. Gold-standard methods for measuring human study data are typically cumbersome, invasive, and expensive, precluding their use in large studies, but such procedures can be performed in smaller groups of people to determine the accuracy of more practical measurement methods. For example, a sample of participants from the study of fish consumption could provide blood samples for the measurement of specific fatty acids derived from fish. These results could be compared with fish consumption reported on the food frequency questionnaires among participants who complete both procedures to estimate the accuracy of the questionnaires.

6.2.2 Are the Measurements Precise?

Precision, or repeatability, refers to how well a measurement returns the same result when performed in succession. For laboratory measurements, such as homocysteine, precision can be assessed by repeating the assay on the same sample and then calculating the degree of inconsistency across the measurements. Similar considerations apply to other exposures, such as blood pressure, which is subject to fluctuation from measurement to measurement. Greater variability in the procedures used to ascertain exposures will generally tend to dilute observed associations with disease. The error caused by imprecision (but not inaccuracy) can be reduced by performing repeated measurements of a study characteristic.

6.2.3 Are the Measurements Applied Impartially to the Study Population?

The procedures used to ascertain study data should ideally be applied consistently to all of the participants in a study. For example, the study of homocysteine levels was conducted at multiple sites within a large health network. An impartial method for measuring this exposure would be to ship all study samples to a central laboratory that performs homocysteine testing. Such procedures avoid the possibility of anomalous results arising from a specific laboratory.

6.2.4 Are the Measurements Performed at the Right Time?

Support for a causal relationship between exposure and disease includes observing associations within a plausible timeframe consistent with knowledge of the disease process. For example, studies reporting an association of cigarette smoking with pneumonia over decades of follow-up are supported by known *long-term* effects of smoking on host defense systems within the lungs. On the other hand, exposure measurements that are ill-timed with the occurrence of disease can sometimes produce spurious associations.

Example 6.6 A cohort study evaluated the association of cigarette smoking with "walking pneumonia," an infection caused by the bacterium *Mycoplasma pneumoniae*. Researchers identified a large cohort of smokers and a large cohort of non-smokers from a community-based health system and followed these cohorts over time for the development of walking pneumonia. Because smoking habits may change over time, the researchers updated the participants' smoking status every 6 months throughout the study via text messaging and email contacts. Paradoxically, the study found current smoking to be associated with a *lower* incidence of walking pneumonia.

Frequently updating smoking status in this study substantially reduces follow-up time between measurement of the exposure and the occurrence of the disease. The study results describe the association between smoking and walking pneumonia over only 6 months, at which time smoking status is again updated. There is no clear mechanistic explanation to support such a short-term impact of smoking on this outcome. One possibility to explain these paradoxical findings is that symptoms of impending pneumonia, such as a productive cough, fever, and malaise, may have prompted some of the smokers in the study to temporarily quit and therefore be classified as "non-smokers" at the time they were diagnosed with the disease. This problem of reverse causality, in which the outcome of a study can itself influence the exposure, is identical to that previously described for cross-sectional studies in Chap. 5.

6.2.5 *Retrospective Versus Prospective Data Collection*

The terms "retrospective" and "prospective" refer to when the study data are collected relative to when the researchers conceive and conduct the study. A retrospective study refers to a study that is conceived after the data have been collected.

Example 6.7 One of the largest cohort studies ever conducted is the Nurses' Health Study, which recruited 127,000 nurses between the ages of 30 and 55 [4]. Beginning in 1976, nurses completed study procedures that assessed medical conditions, surgeries, medication use, social habits, dietary patterns, and physical activity levels. Nurses were followed for over 30 years for the development of major disease outcomes, including diabetes, heart disease, and cancer.

One follow-up study using Nurses' Health Study data evaluated whether coffee consumption is associated with the development of type II diabetes (Example 3.2). This study is "retrospective" in that the researchers conceived and conducted the study after the Nurses' Health Study data had already been collected. Nonetheless, the study design proceeds forward over time: first excluding nurses who had diabetes at the start of the study, next assessing the amount of coffee consumption among diabetes-free nurses from the dietary data, and then determining new cases of diabetes through 1998. A prospective study to address the same question would require the collection of original study data. The distinction between retrospective and prospective studies is generally descriptive and has minimal impact on the interpretation of study results.

6.3 Pharmacoepidemiology Studies

The definitive method for determining the benefits and harms of medications or procedures is to conduct randomized trials, which can separate the effects of these treatments from the characteristics of the people who receive them. However, randomized trials are often conducted among relatively healthy people under controlled conditions, potentially masking the real-world impact of the study treatments. Observational studies of the consequences of medications and procedures, also called *pharmacoepidemiology studies*, can supplement the results obtained from randomized trials by evaluating these treatments in diverse populations under realistic conditions. Pharmacoepidemiology studies have the potential to identify uncommon and unintended side effects of approved medications that may be missed in clinical trials [5]. For example, peroxisome proliferator-activated receptor (PPAR) agonists are medications used to control blood sugars in patients with type II diabetes. Initial trials demonstrated that these medications reduced levels of glycosylated hemoglobin, a marker of blood sugar control. Longer-term observational studies that assessed large numbers of PPAR agonist users and nonusers were needed to recognize that these drugs paradoxically *increased* the risk of coronary heart disease.

Pharmacoepidemiology studies can also be useful for appraising the values and harms of medications in vulnerable populations that are likely to be excluded from trials, such as pregnant women or patients who have advanced liver or kidney disease.

Example 6.8 Selective serotonin reuptake inhibitors (SSRIs) are among the most commonly prescribed antidepressant medications. SSRIs are frequently used during pregnancy; however, the impact of these drugs on fetal development is uncertain. A cohort study identified 36,778 women who used SSRIs during the first trimester of pregnancy and a comparison group of 180,564 pregnant women who also had a diagnosis of depression but did not use SSRIs [6]. The study found low and nearly identical rates of fetal cardiac malformations among these groups.

This study obtained important safety information regarding SSRIs that could not be easily obtained from trials, because randomized trials frequently exclude pregnant women due to concerns regarding safety and because trials could not feasibly evaluate such a large number of women needed to assess this relatively uncommon outcome.

As with other types of observational studies, the primary limitation of pharmacoepidemiology studies is the possibility of bias arising from potential differences in the characteristics of exposed versus unexposed people (confounding). The study of SSRI use and cardiac malformations carefully measured and adjusted for many characteristics that may have differed between pregnant women who used SSRIs and those who did not. However, differences in unmeasured characteristics may have distorted the study findings. A second potential limitation of pharmacoepidemiology studies is called *prevalent user bias*. This problem can arise in studies that preferentially evaluate long-standing users of a particular medication, thereby potential missing early adverse effects of the drug. For example, estrogen treatment can abruptly increase the risk of venous thromboembolism (blood clot) among women who have a genetic susceptibility to clotting. Previous observational studies of estrogen use tended to focus on long-term users, potentially missing acute thromboembolic events that would have prompted early termination of this treatment. Prevalent user bias can be avoided by evaluating medication use at the time of first initiation, analogous to the approach used in randomized trials.

6.4   Analysis of Cohort Study Data

6.4.1   Calculation of Disease Incidences Among the Cohorts

The fundamental analysis in cohort studies is to compare the incidence of disease among the cohorts. Consider data from the fictitious study of antibiotic use and rash (Example 6.3), shown in Table 6.1.

Recall that incidence proportion is defined as the number of new cases of a disease that develop over time divided by the number of people who are initially free of the disease. Presuming that participants in the antibiotic study were free of rash at the start of the study:

$$\text{Incidence proportion of rash}\left(\text{supramycin users}\right) = \frac{10\,\text{new rashes}}{100\,\text{initially free of rash}} \overset{*}{} 100\%$$
$$= 10\%$$

$$\text{Incidence proportion of rash}\left(\text{amoxicillin users}\right) = \frac{20\,\text{new rashes}}{400\,\text{initially free of rash}} \overset{*}{} 100\%$$
$$= 5\%$$

If person-time data are available, incidence rates provide a more accurate comparison of disease occurrence than incidence proportions. Given total follow-up times of 170 weeks in the supramycin group and 720 weeks in the amoxicillin group, the incidence rates of rash would be:

$$\text{Incidence rate of rash}\left(\text{supramycin users}\right) = \frac{10\,\text{new rashes}}{170\,\text{person} - \text{weeks}}$$
$$= 5.9\,\text{rashes}\,/\,100\,\text{person} - \text{weeks}$$

$$\text{Incidence rate of rash}\left(\text{amoxicillin users}\right) = \frac{20\,\text{new rashes}}{720\,\text{person} - \text{weeks}}$$
$$= 2.8\,\text{rashes}\,/\,100\,\text{person} - \text{weeks}$$

Table 6.1 Hypothetical cohort study of antibiotic use and rash

	Rash		
	Yes	No	Total
Supramycin use	10	90	100
Amoxicillin use	20	380	400
Total	30	470	500

6.4.2   Comparison of Disease Incidences Among the Cohorts

6.4.2.1   Relative Risk

The most straightforward expression that compares disease incidences is relative risk.

$$\text{Relative risk} = \text{Incidence}\left(\text{exposed cohort}\right)/\text{Incidence}\left(\text{unexposed cohort}\right)$$

The relative risk of rash, comparing supramycin use to amoxicillin use, can be calculated from the incidence rate data provided above.

$$\text{Relative risk} = \frac{\text{Incidence exposed}}{\text{Incidence unexposed}} = \frac{5.9\,\text{rashes per}\,100\,\text{person} - \text{weeks}}{2.8\,\text{rashes per}\,100\,\text{person} - \text{weeks}}$$
$$= 2.11\left(\text{no units}\right)$$

This relative risk can be interpreted as, "supramycin use is associated with a 2.11-times greater risk of rash compared to amoxicillin use." An equally correct interpretation of this relative risk would be, "supramycin use is associated with a 111% greater risk of rash compared to amoxicillin use." The "111% greater" risk derives from the fact that 2.11 is "111% greater" than the value of 1.0 that would be observed if no association was present.

The designation of supramycin users as the exposed cohort demonstrates relative harm associated with the use of this antibiotic, in terms of rash. Alternatively, the selection of amoxicillin users as the exposed cohort reorients the study results in terms of characteristics that might prevent, rather than cause, a rash.

$$\text{Relative risk} = \frac{\text{Incidence unexposed}}{\text{Incidence exposed}} = \frac{2.8\,\text{rashes per}\,100\,\text{person} - \text{weeks}}{5.9\,\text{rashes per}\,100\,\text{person} - \text{weeks}}$$
$$= 0.47\left(\text{no units}\right)$$

This relative risk can be interpreted as, "amoxicillin use is associated with a 53% lower risk of rash compared to supramycin use." The "53% lower" derives from the fact that 0.47 is 53% lower than the unity value of 1.0 that would be observed if no association was present.

Why is supramycin use associated with a 111% greater risk of rash, but amoxicillin use associated with only a 53% lower risk of rash? In other words, why are the relative risks not symmetrical for the same exposure? Relative risks, like all ratios, can assume possible values ranging from 0 to infinity; however, 1.0 defines the unity value. It is more difficult to obtain relative risks that are much less than 1.0 because they are bounded at 0. For this reason, relative risks less than 1.0 indicate stronger associations than symmetrical associations greater than 1.0.

The relative risks described above do not address the possibility that supramycin users may differ from amoxicillin users by other characteristics that could predis-

Table 6.2 Association of serum homocysteine levels with peripheral arterial disease

Serum homocysteine level (umol/L)	Number of participants	Peripheral arterial disease events during follow-up	Person-years	Incidence rate[a]
<15	1200	8	4560	1.8
15–30	2600	28	9620	2.9
31–100	1800	24	6570	3.7
>100	1200	36	3840	9.4

[a]Incidence rates expressed as number of events per 1000 person-years

pose to rash, such as older age or a previous history of drug allergy. Procedures to adjust relative risks for differences in participant characteristics are discussed in Chap. 10. Relative risks that are calculated using only the raw study data, such as those calculated above, are often termed "unadjusted" or "crude" relative risks to denote the lack of adjustment.

How are relative risks calculated for studies with more than two cohorts? For example, the study of serum homocysteine levels and peripheral arterial disease may divide this exposure into four mutually exclusive categories, shown in Table 6.2.

To obtain relative risks for a study with multiple cohorts, one cohort must be designated as the *reference cohort*. As with the choice of exposed and unexposed cohorts, the selection of a reference group is flexible and depends on the study question. In this example, the implicit hypothesis is that higher homocysteine levels are associated with greater risks of peripheral arterial disease, motivating designation of the lowest homocysteine category as the reference group. Relative risks can then be calculated for each cohort in relation to the reference cohort:

Cohort	Incidence rate	Relative risk
Homocysteine <15 umol/L	1.8	*Reference group*
Homocysteine 15–30 umol/L	2.9	2.9/1.8 = 1.6
Homocysteine 31–100 umol/L	3.7	3.7/1.8 = 2.1
Homocysteine >100 umol/L	9.4	9.4/1.8 = 5.2

The relative risk for the highest serum homocysteine category would be interpreted as, "serum homocysteine levels >100 umol/L are associated with a 5.2-times greater incidence of peripheral arterial disease compared with levels <15 umol/L." The reference group should be included in this statement because it is fundamental to the definition of relative risk. Of note, many research articles designate the reference cohort using a relative risk of 1.0 with no corresponding confidence interval or p-value.

Some cohort studies use graphical methods to present risks for continuous exposures. For example, researchers in the homocysteine study could plot measured homocysteine levels on the X-axis versus the incidence of peripheral arterial disease on the Y-axis and then calculate the slope, shown in Fig. 6.3.

In this instance, risk is not reported in relation to any specific reference group but is applicable to a given difference in levels of the exposure. Based on the estimated

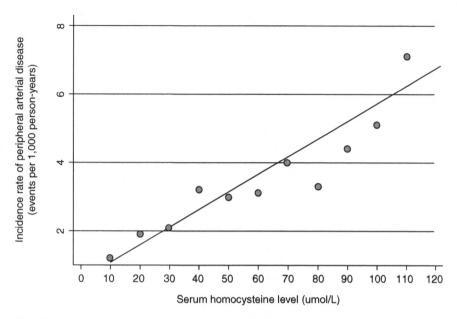

Fig. 6.3 Association of continuous homocysteine levels with peripheral arterial disease

slope in Fig 6.3, each 20 umol/L higher serum homocysteine level is associated with an approximate 1.0 event per 1000 person-years higher incidence of peripheral arterial disease. Stated another way, a person with a serum homocysteine level of 70 umol/L has an incidence of peripheral arterial disease that is 1.0 per 1,000 person-years higher compared with a person with a serum homocysteine level of 50 umol/L. The figure provides important information regarding an exposure-varying association between the exposure and outcome.

6.4.2.2 Attributable Risk

Relative risks have a comparatively straightforward interpretation that can be applied to individuals. The relative risk for the highest serum homocysteine category in Table 6.2 can be interpreted as, "a *person* with a serum homocysteine level >100 umol/L has a 5.2-times greater incidence of peripheral arterial disease than a *person* with a serum homocysteine level <15 umol/L." Other comparisons of incidences, including attributable risk and population attributable risk, describe the impact of an exposure on a population of interest. The interpretation of these measures assumes a reasonable degree of certainty that the exposure itself is likely causing the observed difference in outcomes. This assumption may be reasonable when interpreting results obtained from large randomized trials, or those obtained from observational studies that are supported by established biological evidence, such as the association of smoking with lung cancer. However, the interpretation of attributable and population attributable risks for nascent observational data is more ambiguous due to the possibility of distortion by potential differences in the characteristics of exposed versus unexposed people (confounding).

Attributable risk, also called *absolute risk reduction*, describes the quantity of additional outcomes among the exposed cohort that is attributable to the exposure.

$$\text{Attributable risk} = \text{Incidence}(\text{exposed cohort}) - \text{Incidence}(\text{unexposed cohort})$$

For the hypothetical study comparing supramycin to amoxicillin for the development of rash:

$$\text{Attributable risk} = \text{Incidence}(\text{supramycin use}) - \text{Incidence}(\text{amoxicillin use})$$
$$= 5.9\,\text{rashes per}\,100\,\text{person-years} - 2.8\,\text{rashes per}\,100 - \text{person years}$$
$$= 3.1\,\text{rashes per}\,100\,\text{person-years}$$

Note that attributable risk, unlike relative risk, maintains the same units as the incidence values. The attributable risk associated with supramycin use is depicted graphically in Fig. 6.4.

If supramycin use itself were the sole cause of the additional rashes observed in this study, then there are 3.1 additional rashes per 100 person-years in the supramycin group that are attributable to the use of this antibiotic.

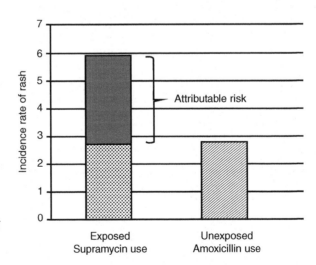

Fig. 6.4 Attributable risk of rash associated with supramycin use

6.4.2.3   Population Attributable Risk

Population attributable risk describes the quantity of additional outcomes in the *total study population* that are attributable to an exposure. Like attributable risk, the interpretation of population attributable risk assumes that the exposure of interest is the exclusive cause of observed differences in disease outcomes.

$$\text{Population attributable risk} = \text{Incidence}\left(\text{total population}\right)$$
$$- \text{Incidence}\left(\text{unexposed cohort}\right)$$

The calculation of population attributable risk requires determination of the disease incidence among the total study population. The overall incidence of rash in the antibiotic study can be calculated from the data in Table 6.1.

$$\text{Incidence rate of rash}\left(\text{total population}\right) = \frac{30\,\text{new rashes}}{890\,\text{person} - \text{weeks}}$$
$$= 3.4\,\text{rashes} / 100\,\text{person} - \text{weeks}$$

$$\text{Population attributable risk} = \text{Incidence}\left(\text{total population}\right)$$
$$- \text{Incidence}\left(\text{amoxicillin use}\right)$$
$$= 3.4\,\text{rashes per 100 person-years} - 2.8\,\text{rashes per 100 person-years}$$
$$= 0.6\,\text{rashes per 100 person-years}$$

The population attributable risk associated with supramycin use is illustrated in Fig. 6.5.

Under the assumption that supramycin use is the sole cause of the additional rashes observed in this study, the population attributable risk can be interpreted as, "there are 0.6 extra rashes per 100 person-years in the population that are attributable to supramycin use." The population in question is persons with pneumonia who receive either supramycin or amoxicillin treatment.

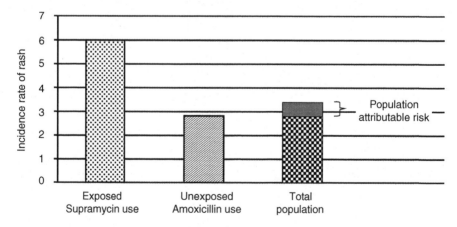

Fig. 6.5 Population attributable risk of rash associated with supramycin use

Population attributable risks can be considered to represent the expected impact of removing a potentially harmful exposure or risk factor from a population. An alternate interpretation of the population attributable risk data would be, "removing the (putatively harmful) supramycin antibiotic from the population would be expected to reduce the rate of rash by 0.6 cases per 100 person-years."

6.4.2.4 Other Measures of Risk

Attributable risk and population attributable risk can be expressed as proportions relative to the exposed and total populations, respectively.

$$\text{Attributable risk percent} = \frac{\left[\text{Incidence}\left(\text{exposed}\right) - \text{Incidence}\left(\text{unexposed}\right)\right]^{*}}{\text{Incidence}\left(\text{exposed}\right)} \; 100\%$$

$$\text{Population attributable risk percent} =$$
$$\frac{\left[\text{Incidence}\left(\text{population}\right) - \text{Incidence}\left(\text{unexposed}\right)\right]^{*}}{\text{Incidence}\left(\text{population}\right)} \; 100\%$$

These measures are used to describe the proportion of outcomes in the exposed population or total population that are expected to be impacted by the exposure.

6.5 Advantages of Cohort Studies

6.5.1 Ability to Discern Temporal Relationships Between Exposure and Disease

Presuming that the study population is truly free of the disease at the time of exposure measurements, cohort studies can discern temporal relationships between potential risk factors and disease outcomes. Demonstration of a temporal association supports the hypothesis that the exposure is a cause of the disease.

6.5.2 Ability to Study Multiple Outcomes

Cohort studies provide the opportunity to study multiple outcomes, efficiently leveraging resources to address broad scientific questions related to population health. For example, the Nurses' Health Study collected comprehensive exposure information among a large group of study participants and then followed them over many years for the development of several important health outcomes. Data from the Nurses' Health Study has been used to investigate a wide range of diseases and risk factors.

6.6   Limitations of Cohort Studies

6.6.1   Confounding

Cohort studies, like other observational study designs, measure exposures that occur "naturally." Consequently, exposed and unexposed individuals may differ by characteristics that could impact the outcomes under study. Confounding defines a type of bias that occurs when characteristics other than the exposure of interest distort or bias the observed association between exposure and disease. The possibility of confounding obscures whether the associations seen observational studies represent causal relationships. The association between the supramycin use and rash could represent the causal impact of this antibiotic on rash but could also be distorted by differences in the characteristics of people who received supramycin compared with those who received amoxicillin. Cohort studies may carefully measure and control for many characteristics that differ between exposed and unexposed individuals. Nonetheless, it is impossible to measure *all* of the characteristics that might be confounding an observed association, leaving residual uncertainty regarding causality.

6.6.2   Inefficient Design for Rare Diseases and Those with a Long Latency Period

Cohort studies are inefficient for studying uncommon diseases and, for prospective studies, diseases that have a long latency period between the exposure and the onset of disease.

Example 6.9 Amyotrophic lateral sclerosis (ALS) is a severe and progressive neurodegenerative disorder. In addition to genetic susceptibility, environmental factors have been postulated to increase the risk of the disease, including exposure to heavy metals such as cadmium. A cohort study to examine whether cadmium, which is used in the production of batteries and alloys, is associated with ALS would be difficult to conduct, because ALS occurs in only about 2 in 100,000 people. Millions of exposed and unexposed workers would need to be studied to demonstrate meaningful differences in the incidence of ALS.

Example 6.10 Childhood epilepsy may be a risk factor for developing migraine headache later in life. Although migraine headache is not a rare outcome, a cohort study to assess this association would be challenging to perform prospectively, due to the long latency period between childhood epilepsy and the occurrence of adult migraine headache.

Rare diseases and those with long latency periods are more efficiently evaluated using a case-control study design, which is described in Chap. 7.

References

1. Kestenbaum B, Rudser KD, de Boer IH, et al. Differences in kidney function and incident hypertension: the multi-ethnic study of atherosclerosis. Ann Intern Med. 2008;148(7):501–8.
2. Bild DE, Bluemke DA, Burke GL, et al. Multi-Ethnic Study of Atherosclerosis: objectives and design. Am J Epidemiol. 2002;156(9):871–81.
3. He K, Xun P, Brasky TM, Gammon MD, Stevens J, White E. Types of fish consumed and fish preparation methods in relation to pancreatic cancer incidence: the VITAL Cohort Study. Am J Epidemiol. 2013;177(2):152–60.
4. Belanger CF, Hennekens CH, Rosner B, Speizer FE. The nurses' health study. Am J Nurs. 1978;78(6):1039–40.
5. Avorn J. In defense of pharmacoepidemiology – embracing the yin and yang of drug research. N Engl J Med. 2007;357(22):2219–21.
6. Hviid A, Melbye M, Pasternak B. Use of selective serotonin reuptake inhibitors during pregnancy and risk of autism. N Engl J Med. 2013;369(25):2406–15.

Chapter 7
Case-Control Studies

Summary of Learning Points

7.1 Case-control studies are observational studies that are conducted in three basic steps:

    7.1.1 Identify people who have a specific disease or condition

    7.1.2 Identify a comparison group of people who do not have this condition

    7.1.3 Determine the proportion of each group who had a previous exposure

7.2 To increase the chance of obtaining valid associations in case-control studies:

    7.2.1 Cases should be selected using a specific definition of the disease.

    7.2.2 Controls should be selected from the same underlying population as the cases.

    7.2.3 Nested case control studies select cases and controls from a unified population.

    7.2.4 Matching may be performed to increase similarity between cases and controls.

    7.2.5 A steep increase in study power is achieved until about 3–4 controls per case.

7.3 Analysis of case-control data

    7.3.1 The odds ratio is the primary measure of association in case-control studies.

    7.3.2 Odds ratios approximate relative risks when the disease outcome is rare.

7.4 Advantages of case-control studies include:

    7.4.1 Useful for studying rare diseases

    7.4.2 Can efficiently determine associations using relatively few study participants

    7.4.3 Can evaluate multiple risk factors for a disease outcome

© Springer Nature Switzerland AG 2019
B. Kestenbaum, *Epidemiology and Biostatistics*,
https://doi.org/10.1007/978-3-319-96644-1_7

7.5 Limitations of case-control studies include:

    7.5.1 Confounding characteristics other than the exposure of interest may bias observed associations with disease

    7.5.2 Valid measurements of previous exposures must be obtained in retrospect

    7.5.3 Study design prohibits direct calculation of the incidence of disease

7.1 Case-Control Study Design

Case-control studies are observational studies that begin by targeting a disease or condition of interest and then work backward to determine associations with previous exposures. The case-control study design is ideally suited for examining potential risk factors for rare diseases.

Consider a new study question: is receipt of the measles-mumps-rubella (MMR) vaccine associated with pervasive developmental disorders, including autism, in children? A hypothetical cohort study to address this question would begin by identifying one group of children who received the MMR vaccine and another group of children who did not receive this vaccine. The cohort study would then follow these children over time to ascertain new occurrences of developmental disorder, shown in Table 7.1.

The hypothetical cohort study evaluated a reasonably large number of children; however, too few cases of pervasive developmental disorder occurred during the study to draw meaningful conclusions regarding a possible link with MMR vaccination.

A case-control study to address the same question would begin by targeting the outcome: pervasive developmental disorder. Such a study would first identify a group of children who had been diagnosed with this condition. *These are the cases.* Next, the study would identify a comparison group of children who did not have a developmental disorder. *These are the controls.* The study would then work backward to determine the proportion of children in each group who had previously undergone MMR vaccination.

In one such case-control study, investigators queried the United Kingdom (UK) General Practice Research Database to identify 1300 children who had received a diagnosis of pervasive developmental disorder [1]. Concurrently, the investigators

Table 7.1 Hypothetical cohort study of MMR vaccine and pervasive developmental disorder

	New cases of developmental disorder		
	Yes	No	Incidence proportion (%)
MMR vaccination (exposed)	8	724	1.1
No MMR vaccination (unexposed)	2	179	1.1

Table 7.2 Case-control study of MMR vaccination and pervasive developmental disorder

	Developmental disorder	
	Yes (cases)	No (controls)
MMR vaccination	1000 (77%)	3550 (79%)
No MMR vaccination	300 (23%)	950 (21%)
Total	1300	4500

selected a comparison group of 4500 control children from the same UK database who did not have a developmental disorder. Study personnel then reviewed the medical records of case and control children to determine their previous MMR vaccination status, shown in Table 7.2.

MMR vaccination was similarly common among the case and control children in the study, suggesting that this vaccine is *not* associated with the occurrence of pervasive developmental disorder. In contrast to the hypothetical cohort study, the case-control study was able to obtain reliable estimates of the proportion of MMR vaccination among children with and without pervasive developmental disorder by directly targeting the disease of interest.

7.2 Selection of Cases and Controls

7.2.1 Select Case Individuals Using a Specific Definition of the Disease

Ideally, case-control studies should select case individuals based on a high degree of certainty for having the disease of interest (case specificity). The inadvertent inclusion of non-diseased people as "cases" can greatly diminish the potential of a case-control study to detect associations. For example, a highly specific definition of pervasive developmental disorder might require the fulfillment of *all* diagnostic criteria for this condition by two highly experienced clinicians. Such a specific definition of the disease may exclude less distinct conditions, such as language-based learning disorders in children, restricting applicability of the study findings to children who have a definitive diagnosis of the disease. However, such a tradeoff is generally preferred in case-control studies due to the importance of ensuring that case individuals truly have the condition of interest. Analogously, a case-control study that examines the association between indoor tanning and melanoma would ideally select cases based on biopsy proven evidence of invasive melanoma, and potentially exclude precancerous lesions, such as dysplastic nevi (mole). On the other hand, it is generally less important for case-control studies to devote extraordinary resources toward confirming that control individuals are free of the disease, because case-control studies typically evaluate rare diseases that are unlikely to be present in otherwise healthy people.

7.2.2   Select Case Individuals Close to the Time of Initial Disease Development

In some instances, the selection of case individuals who *recently* developed the disease greatly facilitates reliable ascertainment of previous exposures. For example, identifying case children who recently received a diagnosis of developmental disorder greatly simplifies ascertainment of previous MMR vaccination status, which may have occurred at the same clinic or healthcare facility. It may be considerably more difficult to determine previous MMR vaccination status in older children or adults with a long-standing diagnosis of developmental disorder.

A second reason for selecting case individuals close to the time of disease onset is to avoid conflating the development of a disease with survivorship.

Example 7.1 A hypothetical case-control study examines the association of heavy alcohol use with dementia. Researchers identify 90 older adults who have an established diagnosis of dementia from chronic nursing facilities. The average duration of dementia among these case individuals is 8 years. The researchers next identify 200 control individuals without a diagnosis of dementia from the same nursing facilities. Study personnel review the medical records of cases and controls to determine previous histories of heavy alcohol use. The study finds that 6% of cases and 6% of controls have a previous history of heavy alcohol use, suggesting no association of this exposure with dementia.

Potential errors in ascertaining alcohol use from medical record data may have contributed to the null findings in this study. However, a second potential limitation is the preferential selection of case individuals who were long-term survivors of dementia. This strategy may have specfically missed rapidly progressive and fatal forms of dementia that can be caused by heavy alcohol use.

7.2.3   Select Control Individuals from the Same Underlying Population as the Cases

The best way to obtain an unbiased estimate of the frequency of past exposures is to select control individuals who were members of the same underlying population as the cases. For example, researchers conducting the study of developmental disorder selected control children who were members of the same UK practice database and were from similar geographic regions as the case children. What if the researchers had instead selected control children from regions that tend to be distrustful of vaccines? Such children may have systematically low levels of MMR vaccination relative to the case children, creating the false appearance of an association between vaccination and developmental disorder. Conversely, preferential selection of control children from clinics that assertively promote vaccination could artificially inflate the frequency of this exposure relative to that of the case children, creating a false association between non-vaccination and developmental disorder.

Example 7.2 A case-control study investigated whether wearing a helmet is associated with a lower risk of serious head injury among skiers and snowboarders [2]. The researchers identified 147 case individuals who suffered a serious head injury while skiing or snowboarding at one of eight Norwegian resorts. Based on ski patrol reports, 17% of the injured skiers and snowboarders were wearing a helmet at the time of their injury. The researchers next attempted to identify a suitable control population that would provide an impartial estimate of the prevalence of helmet use among non-injured skiers and snowboarders.

It may not be possible to obtain an unequivocally representative control group. The researchers elected to interview well-appearing (non-injured) skiers and snowboarders who were waiting in the lift lines at the same resorts. They selected the busiest times of the day and chose lifts that covered a wide variety of terrain and difficulty levels. Nonetheless, it remains possible that this procedure overestimated or underestimated the true frequency of helmet use in the larger population of skiers and snowboarders from whom the injured cases arose.

7.2.4 Select Control Individuals Who Have the Same Opportunity to Be Counted as a Case

Case-control studies typically evaluate rare diseases, which may be identified from registries, pathology databases, hospital records, or other specialized sources. Control individuals selected for these studies should have access to the same procedures for disease detection as the cases. For example, a case-control study of mesothelioma, a rare form of lung cancer, identified case patients from a cancer registry in the Pacific Northwest that receives data from hospitals, oncologists, pathologists, and radiotherapists. Controls for this study were selected from healthcare facilities that report to this same cancer registry to ensure that they *would have been counted as a case* had they developed mesothelioma during the study.

7.2.5 Nested Case-Control Studies

A formal method to certify that case and control individuals are selected from the same underlying population is a nested case-control study. Such studies identify cases and controls from within a larger unified study population, such as a cohort study.

Example 7.3 The Multi-Ethnic Study of Atherosclerosis (MESA) is a prospective cohort study of 6814 adults who were initially free of cardiovascular disease. Participants were followed over 15 years for the development of cardiovascular outcomes. In one nested case-control study, researchers selected 112 case participants from MESA who developed heart failure during the study and a control population of 224 age- and-sex matched MESA participants who did not develop heart failure during this same time period [3]. The researchers analyzed cardiac imaging data that were initially obtained at the start of MESA to determine associations of left atrial functions with incident heart failure.

This case-control study is *nested* within the larger MESA cohort study and satisfies the previously described criteria for case and control selection. First, incident heart failure events that occurred during MESA were validated by physician adjudication of medical record data, providing a highly specific definition of the disease outcome. Second, heart failure cases were selected close to the time of disease onset, because MESA participants were initially free of cardiovascular diseases, including heart failure, at the start of the study. Third, case and control participants were selected from the same underlying MESA cohort study population. Fourth, controls were followed prospectively in MESA using identical study procedures as the cases, providing an equal opportunity for controls to be diagnosed with heart failure if the disease had occurred.

7.2.6 Matching

Matching can be used in case-control studies to increase the degree of similarity in one or more characteristics between the cases and controls. Given appropriate analysis of the matched study data, matching can reduce the possibility that characteristics other than exposure of interest may be distorting an observed association with disease. For example, researchers in the MESA heart failure study matched each case participant who developed heart failure to two control participants who did not develop heart failure by age (within 5 years) and sex. Table 7.3 demonstrates matching as an iterative process for the first three case participants in this study.

Table 7.3 Matching two controls per case by age and sex

Case individuals (developed heart failure)		Matched control individuals (did not develop heart failure)			
		Control one		Control two	
Age	Sex	Age	Sex	Age	Sex
64	Male	62	Male	65	Male
58	Female	60	Female	61	Female
72	Female	69	Female	74	Female
And so on...					

Repeating this procedure will create a study population in which the mean age and the proportions of men and women will be similar among the cases and controls.

Matching characteristics in case-control studies should include those that themselves are risk factors for the disease but are not consequences of the exposure of interest. In this instance, age and sex are established risk factors for heart failure, based on knowledge from previous studies, but are not consequences of left atrial enlargement or cardiac function. It is possible for matching to artificially dilute associations if this procedure is performed on potential mechanisms that can link the exposure with the disease. For example, greater left atrial size may promote the development of atrial fibrillation, a cardiac arrhythmia that can subsequently increase the risk of heart failure. In other words, atrial fibrillation represents a potential mechanism linking greater left atrial size with heart failure. Matching heart failure cases to non-heart failure controls by the presence of atrial fibrillation could create a false degree of similarity in left atrial size between these groups and mask associations of this exposure with heart failure.

7.2.7   Number of Controls

Finding cases is often the rate-limiting step in case-control studies, because such studies tend to focus on rare diseases. There are no specific rules regarding the size of the control population; study resources often dictate the number of controls that can be selected per case. A greater number of controls will provide a more reliable estimate of the frequency of the exposure and can increase study power (the ability to detect associations that are truly present). There is a steep increase in power as more controls are added until reaching about three to four controls per case, at which point adding more controls has little further effect.

7.3   Analysis of Case Control Study Data

7.3.1   Concept of the Odds Ratio

The analysis of case-control study data differs from that of cohort studies due to the fundamental difference in how participants are selected for these studies. Cohort studies identify groups of exposed and unexposed people and then follow them over time to contrast their incidence of disease. Case-control studies select groups of diseased and non-diseased people and then look backward to measure and compare the proportions who had one or more previous exposures. Consider data from the case-control study of pervasive developmental disorder, shown in Table 7.4.

Table 7.4 Case-control study of MMR vaccination and pervasive developmental disorder

	Developmental disorder	
	Yes (cases)	No (controls)
MMR vaccination	1000	3550
No MMR vaccination	300	950
Total	1300	4500

Table 7.5 Case-control study of developmental disorder with 1300 control children

	Developmental disorder	
	Yes (cases)	No (controls)
MMR vaccination	1000	1027
No MMR vaccination	300	273
Total	1300	1300

Imagine for a moment that these data were collected from a cohort study. Under a cohort study design, the incidence of developmental disorder in each group would be calculated as:

$$\text{``Incidence proportion''}\left(\text{MMR vaccination}\right) = 1000 \,/\, \left(1000 + 3550\right) = 22.0\%$$

$$\text{``Incidence proportion''}\left(\text{No MMR vaccination}\right) = 300 \,/\, \left(300 + 950\right) = 24.0\%$$

However, these calculations represent *false measurements* of disease incidence when the data are obtained from a case-control study, because the frequency of disease in the study is determined by the relative size of the control population. What if the researchers had instead selected only one control child per case, shown in Table 7.5?

$$\text{``Incidence proportion''}\left(\text{MMR vaccination}\right) = 1000 \,/\, \left(1000 + 1027\right) = 49.3\%$$

$$\text{``Incidence proportion''}\left(\text{No MMR vaccination}\right) = 300 \,/\, \left(300 + 273\right) = 52.3\%$$

These (false) incidences are implausibly high for pervasive development disorder, a rare condition previously reported to have an incidence of approximately 1% in the population. These examples demonstrate that *case-control study data, which consist of fixed numbers of people with and without a specific condition of interest, cannot be used to directly obtain valid measurements of incidence.*

The case-control data *can* be used to determine the prevalence of past exposures. Based on the data in Table 7.4:

$$\text{Prevalence of MMR vaccination}\left(\text{cases}\right) = 1000 \,/\, \left(1000 + 300\right) = 76.9\%$$

$$\text{Prevalence of MMR vaccination}\left(\text{controls}\right) = 3550 \,/\, \left(3550 + 950\right) = 78.9\%$$

Table 7.6 Case-control study of pervasive developmental disorder with inflation factor

	Developmental disorder	
	Yes (cases)	No (controls)
MMR vaccination	1000	3550 * X
No MMR vaccination	300	950 * X

Unfortunately, information regarding the frequency of previous exposures has little intrinsic value and is typically unhelpful for informing clinical decisions. The fact that 77% of children who already have a diagnosis of a pervasive developmental disorder previously received the MMR vaccine is not directly helpful for physicians or parents. What is needed is the probability of pervasive developmental disorder comparing children who received the MMR vaccine to those who did not receive this vaccine. This information can be *estimated* from case-control study data through a measure called the *odds ratio*. To develop the concept of the odds ratio, imagine that the control population of the case-control study could be inflated by some factor, "*X*," shown in Table 7.6.

For example, if *X* were equal to 100, then the frequency of pervasive developmental disorder in the case-control study population would be similar to the 1% incidence of this condition previously reported in the population. However, selecting such a large number of control children would be unrealistic. Given that the value of *X* is typically unknown, it is impossible to directly calculate the incidence of developmental disorder among MMR vaccinated or non-vaccinated children from the case-control data alone. However, if the value of *X* is similar in each group, then it *is possible to estimate the ratio of the incidences*, or the *relative risk*, of pervasive developmental disorder, comparing MMR vaccinated to non-vaccinated children:

$$\text{Incidence of developmental disorder}\left(\text{MMR vaccination}\right) \approx 1000 / \left(3550^{*} X\right)$$

$$\text{Incidence of developmental disorder}\left(\text{no MMR vaccination}\right) \approx 1300 / \left(950^{*} X\right)$$

$$\text{Relative risk} = \frac{\text{Incidence exposed}}{\text{Incidence unexposed}} \approx \frac{1000 / \left(3550^{*} X\right)}{300 / \left(950^{*} X\right)}$$

$$\approx \frac{1000 \ / 3550}{300 / 950} \approx 0.89 \left(\text{no units}\right)$$

In other words, the incidence of pervasive developmental disorder among MMR-vaccinated children is *not* 1000/3500 nor is the incidence of pervasive developmental disorder among non-vaccinated children 300/950. However, these false incidences can be regarded as similarly incorrect, such that their ratio approximates the relative risk. The calculated ratio of 0.89 is not exactly a relative risk, which requires a cohort study or advanced methods to calculate directly. Instead, this value represents an estimate of the relative risk and has a different name, the *odds ratio*. *The odds ratio is the principal measure of risk in case-control studies*. Equally correct interpretations of the odds ratio of 0.89 include:

- The odds ratio of pervasive developmental disorder is 0.89, comparing children who previously received the MMR vaccine to those who did not receive this vaccine.
- Previous MMR vaccination is associated with an 11% lower odds of pervasive developmental disorder compared with no MMR vaccination.

The term "odds" is used instead of "risk" in these interpretations to reflect the distinction between the odds ratio and relative risk. Note that the procedure used to estimate relative risk from case-control study data *cannot* be applied to the calculation of attributable risk or population attributable risk, because these measures require *subtracting* the incidences of disease, which are unknown. There is no direct way to calculate attributable risk or population attributable risk from case-control study data alone.

7.3.2   Practical Calculation of the Odds Ratio

The odds ratio can be easily calculated from case-control data using cross multiplication. This procedure requires tabulating the study data as disease versus no disease in the columns of the table and exposure versus no exposure in the rows, shown in Table 7.7.

$$\text{Odds ratio} = \left(a^*d\right)/\left(b^*c\right) = \left(1000^*950\right)/\left(3500^*300\right) = 0.89$$

Note that cross multiplication utilizes raw numbers of people in the cells, not proportions.

7.3.3   Odds Ratios and Relative Risk

Odds ratios provide an estimate of the relative risk of disease associated with an exposure. The agreement between the odds ratio and the relative risk depends on the probability of the disease in the theoretically infinite underlying population from

Table 7.7 Cross multiplication to calculate the odds ratio

	Disease (developmental disorder)	No disease (no developmental disorder)
Exposed (MMR vaccine)	1,000 (a)	3,550 (b)
Unexposed (no MMR vaccine)	300 (c)	950 (d)

which cases and control individuals were drawn. Such information requires knowledge from other studies.

Mathematically, the odds of a disease is defined from disease probability as:

$$\text{Odds} = p / (1 - p)$$

where p represents the probability of a disease in the underlying population. For rare diseases with low probabilities, the denominator, $(1 - p)$, approaches 1.0 and the odds approaches p. On the other hand, odds and probabilities diverge for more common diseases.

Consider a hypothetical risk factor that is associated with a two-fold greater incidence of a disease in the population. A sufficiently large cohort study would calculate a relative risk of approximately 2.0 for this risk factor. In contrast, the odds ratio calculated from a case-control study of this same risk factor would depend on the overall probability of the disease in the underlying population, shown in Table 7.8.

The odds ratio progressively exaggerates the relative risks of more common diseases. However, because most case-control studies examine rare diseases, large distortions are uncommon.

Based on previous studies, the incidence of pervasive developmental disorder is approximately 1% in the population. Therefore, the calculated odds ratio of 0.89, comparing MMR vaccinated to non-MMR vaccinated children, is expected to approximate the relative risk. Consequently, it is permissible to replace the term "odds" with the term "risk" when interpreting this odds ratio to yield a more easily understood result: "Previous MMR vaccination is associated with an 11% lower *risk* of pervasive developmental disorder compared with no MMR vaccination."

On the other hand, case-control studies of more common conditions, such as hypertension, should maintain the term "odds" in their interpretation, because this measure may not approximate the relative risk. The interpretation of odds ratios obtained from case-control studies of common conditions is less straightforward due to the nonintuitive scale of odds.

Importantly, the rare disease assumption applies to the relationship between the odds ratio and the relative risk. *The inability of case-control studies to directly determine the incidence of disease among exposed and unexposed persons is an inherent limitation of this study design and unrelated to the probability of the disease in the population.*

Table 7.8 Agreement between the odds ratio and the relative risk

Probability of disease in the underlying population (%)	Relative risk obtained from a cohort study	Odds ratio obtained from a case-control study
1	2.0	2.02
5	2.0	2.11
10	2.0	2.25
30	2.0	3.50
40	2.0	6.00

Example 7.4 The professional behavior of medical students, including responsibility, self-initiative, and self-improvement, is suggested to be carried forward into their role as physicians. A case-control study investigated the potential consequences of unprofessional behavior during medical school by determining the association with future disciplinary action by a state medical board [4]. Such action is an unusual and serious occurrence that can result from drug or alcohol abuse, negligent professional behavior, or worse. The researchers selected 235 case physicians who had been disciplined by a state medical board and 469 control physicians who had not been disciplined. The researchers then obtained previous medical school records of all study physicians to identify documented episodes of unprofessional behaviors. The study found that a single episode of unprofessional behavior during medical school was associated with an estimated three times greater odds of future disciplinary action by a state medical board.

Several aspects of this study deserve comment. First, the case-control design is ideal for evaluating the outcome of interest, because disciplinary action by a state medical board is rare. A cohort study would require extremely large numbers of physicians to observe enough cases of disciplinary action for valid comparison. Second, the researchers were able to ascertain the exposure, unprofessional behavior during medical school, in retrospect using previously collected data. Had medical school records not been available, the researchers may have been forced to interview the study physicians to assess previous episodes of unprofessional behavior, potentially leading to errors in classifying this exposure. Third, the rarity of disciplinary action by a state medical board permits replacement of the term "odds" with the more easily interpretable term "risk," such that the results of the study can be stated more practically as, "an episode of unprofessional behavior during medical school is associated with a 3-times greater *risk* of incurring disciplinary action by a state medical board."

Nonetheless, the case-control study design precludes direct calculation of the incidence of disciplinary action by a state medical board among medical students who are cited for unprofessional behavior and those who are not. The results of this study demonstrate only that a student who is cited for unprofessional behavior during medical school is about three times more likely to incur future disciplinary action *relative to his/her classmate who is not cited for such behavior*. The probability of disciplinary action by a state medical board is exceeding low for both students and may not be particularly useful for guiding decisions regarding individual students.

7.4 Advantages of Case Control Studies

7.4.1 *Ideal for Studying Rare Diseases and Those with a Long Latency Period*

Case-control studies are ideally suited for investigating underlying causes of uncommon conditions, such as outbreaks of atypical infectious diseases, unpredicted adverse effects of medications, and congenital abnormalities. The case-control design is also commonly applied to studies of genetic causes of common diseases. For example, a case-control study examined genetic determinants of asthma among more than 10,000 children and young adults with an asthma diagnosis and a large control population without asthma. The researchers measured a large array of genetic polymorphisms in the cases and controls to identify inherited variants that were associated with this disease. Although asthma is not rare, the case-control design provides an efficient method for determining associations by concentrating the genotyping procedures on people with established disease and a small fraction of possible controls.

Case-control studies are also useful for evaluating potential risk factors that may cause disease over a long latency period, provided that reliable information regarding these risk factors can be obtained in retrospect. For example, testicular cancer occurs most frequently in younger men, suggesting that prenatal or early-life characteristics might play a causal role. In one case-control study, researchers identified 1645 men who were diagnosed with testicular cancer and a control group of 4445 men who did not have cancer [5]. The researchers then linked cases and controls to state birth record data to obtain information regarding gestational age, birth weight, and parity. A prospective cohort study to test whether these characteristics are associated with testicular cancer would require years-decades of follow-up.

7.4.2   Efficiency

Case-control studies can efficiently determine associations using fewer participants than cohort studies, thereby conserving study resources. Consider the case-control study of heart failure nested within the larger MESA cohort study (Example 7.3). The researchers performed detailed analyses of cardiac imaging data in the 112 participants who developed heart failure and a selected group of 224 control participants who did not develop heart failure to demonstrate an association of left atrial enlargement with this disease. A cohort study to examine this association would require analysis of imagining data from the entire MESA population, which would be expensive and time-consuming. The random sample of controls provided a reasonable estimate of the frequency of left atrial enlargement among all possible MESA controls, shown in Table 7.9.

Table 7.9 Left atrial enlargement among cases, all possible controls, and sample of controls

| | Complete MESA cohort study | | Sample of controls |
	Developed heart failure	Did not develop heart failure	Did not develop heart failure
Number of participants	112	6700	224
Left atrial enlargement	40 (36%)	1340 (20%)	47 (21%)

Table 7.10 Baseline characteristics of heart failure cases and controls

	Developed heart failure	Did not develop heart failure
Number of participants	112	224
Systolic blood pressure (mmHg)	138.4	130.5
Body mass index (kg/m^2)	29.1	27.6
Current smoking (%)	19	11
Diabetes (%)	30	14

7.4.3   Evaluation of Multiple Exposures

Case-control studies can investigate multiple risk factors for a disease within defined groups of cases and controls. Table 7.10 presents some additional exposures in relation to heart failure status in the MESA study.

These data demonstrate higher systolic blood pressure and body mass index, and a higher prevalence of current smoking and diabetes among the cases, suggesting associations of these characteristics with heart failure.

7.5   Limitations of Case Control Studies

7.5.1   Confounding

As a type of observational study, case-control studies evaluate exposures that occur "naturally." Consequently, case-control studies can detect associations between potential risk factors and disease but may fall short of leading to an inference that a risk factor is a *cause* of the disease. For example, the case-control study of skiers and snowboarders from Example 7.2 found that helmet use was associated with a 60% lower odds of sustaining a serious head injury. This association is (clearly) supported by biological plausibility. Nonetheless, it remains possible that other attributes of helmeted skiers and snowboarders, such as more cautious skiing habits, may have also contributed to the observed lower risk of injury. Observational studies, including case-control and cohort studies, strive to minimize confounding by measuring and adjusting for characteristics that can bias the study results but may not be able to account for all possible confounding factors.

7.5.2   Requires Ascertainment of Previous Exposures in Retrospect

The ability of case-control studies to produce valid associations depends on the ability to obtain valid measurements of previous exposures in retrospect. In some instances, accurate data regarding past exposures can be ascertained from preexisting records, such as medical charts, birth registries, telephone records, or radiology reports. If information regarding previous exposures cannot be obtained from existing sources, then researchers conducting case-control studies may be forced to directly interview participants to obtain these data.

Example 7.5   A case-control study evaluated potential risk factors for HIV seroconversion among healthcare workers who had an occupational exposure to HIV-infected blood. Case individuals were 33 healthcare workers who became HIV seropositive following a needle stick injury from an HIV positive patient. Control individuals were 665 healthcare workers who were also exposed to HIV-positive blood but remained HIV seronegative. Characteristics that were suspected to impact the risk of seroconversion included the depth of the needle stick injury, the size of the needle, and whether gloves were worn at the time of injury. How should these exposures be ascertained in retrospect?

Researchers conducting this study obtained exposure data from incident reports required by hospital policy immediately after an occupational needle stick injury. Some errors in ascertaining the details of the needle stick injuries may have occurred due to reliance on participant's recollection of events. Nonetheless, the collection of exposure data promptly following the needle stick likely facilitated the accuracy of these measurements. Importantly, the exposure data were collected before the participants were aware of their subsequent HIV seroconversion status.

If incident reports had not been not available, then the researchers may have been forced to interview case and control individuals to obtain information regarding the needle stick injury. One problem with this approach is that the accuracy of recollection may be compromised by the long period of time since the injury occurred. General errors in measuring attributes of the needle stick injury will typically dilute associations of these characteristics with HIV seroconversion.

Of potentially greater concern is the possibility of systematic error arising from differential recollection of events among case and control individuals. *Recall bias* describes a specific type of bias that can occur in case-control studies when case or control individuals preferentially distort their reporting of previous exposures. For example, healthcare workers who seroconverted (cases) are likely to know they have contracted a serious disease. Such knowledge may impact their recollection and description of the details surrounding the needle stick injury, such as overemphasizing the depth of the injury to find a reason for their illness, or withholding information about wearing gloves due to feelings of guilt. Recall bias can produce opposing distortions of exposure frequencies between cases and controls with a wide range of possible impacts on the study findings, including exaggerating the size of the observed association, diluting the association, or creating false associations. This potential problem can be eliminated by ascertaining previous exposures from sources created prior to the occurrence of the disease. For instances in which interviews are necessary to ascertain previous exposures, the researchers may attempt to conceal specific exposure of interest to minimize the possibility of recall bias.

Example 7.6 Vasculitis is a rare group of autoimmune disorders that cause damage to blood vessels, lungs, and other organ systems. Some preliminary data suggests that the inhalation of silica dust may play a role in the development of this disease. To pursue this hypothesis, researchers identified 126 case individuals who had a biopsy-confirmed dagnosis of vasculitis from hospitals in North Carolina, South Carolina, Georgia, and Virginia and a group of 109 control individuals who did not have a diagnosis of vasculitis from the same geographic regions [6]. During structured interviews, the researchers obtained detailed employment histories, including the type, duration, and location of previous jobs, but did not specifically mention silica. The researchers then estimated silica exposure based on the occupational histories.

Recall bias could still have occurred in this study if case individuals, who were likely aware of their vasculitis diagnosis, preferentially distorted their previous employment histories relative to the controls. Nonetheless, the study procedures attempted to reduce recall bias by concealing the primary exposure of interest.

7.5.3   Inability to Directly Determine the Incidence of Disease

The procedures used to select case and control individuals preclude direct calculation of the incidence of disease among exposed or unexposed individuals. The case-control study of vasculitis cannot directly determine the incidence of this disease among people who have an occupational exposure to silica dust or those who are not exposed to silica. The case-control data can be used to estimate the relative risk of vasculitis comparing people with differing levels of silica exposure. These results can be considered in context with data from other studies to infer a possible causal role of silica exposure in the disease process.

References

1. Smeeth L, Cook C, Fombonne E, et al. MMR vaccination and pervasive developmental disorders: a case-control study. Lancet. 2004;364(9438):963–9.
2. Sulheim S, Holme I, Ekeland A, Bahr R. Helmet use and risk of head injuries in alpine skiers and snowboarders. JAMA. 2006;295(8):919–24.
3. Habibi M, Chahal H, Opdahl A, et al. Association of CMR-measured LA function with heart failure development: results from the MESA study. JACC Cardiovasc Imaging. 2014;7(6):570–9.
4. Papadakis MA, Teherani A, Banach MA, et al. Disciplinary action by medical boards and prior behavior in medical school. N Engl J Med. 2005;353(25):2673–82.
5. English PB, Goldberg DE, Wolff C, Smith D. Parental and birth characteristics in relation to testicular cancer risk among males born between 1960 and 1995 in California (United States). Cancer Causes Control. 2003;14(9):815–25.
6. Hogan SL, Cooper GS, Savitz DA, et al. Association of silica exposure with anti-neutrophil cytoplasmic autoantibody small-vessel vasculitis: a population-based, case-control study. Clin J Am Soc Nephrol. 2007;2(2):290–9.

Chapter 8
Randomized Trials

Summary of Learning Points

8.1 Randomized trials should be considered when there is ongoing uncertainty regarding the impact of a treatment.

8.2 Randomized trials are prospective studies that assess outcomes that occur over time.

8.3 Several considerations inform selection of the study population in randomized trials:

8.3.1 Pragmatic definition of the target condition increases applicability of trial results.

8.3.2 Common exclusion criteria include suspected nonadherence, comorbid diseases, current use of the study treatments, and presumed harm from treatment.

8.4 Randomized trials assign participants to study treatments versus control procedures.

8.4.1 The intervention can be any form of treatment or the target of a treatment.

8.4.2 The comparison group can receive a placebo, a similar treatment, delayed treatment, an accepted standard of care, or no treatment at all.

8.5 Ideal trial outcomes should capture the multidimensional impacts of the interventions.

8.5.1 Trial outcomes should be measured with a high degree of certainty.

8.5.2 Surrogate endpoints are characteristics that change in response to treatment in a manner consistent with the anticipated clinical impact of that treatment.

8.6 Randomization, blinding, and concealment are used to increase internal validity.

© Springer Nature Switzerland AG 2019
B. Kestenbaum, *Epidemiology and Biostatistics*,
https://doi.org/10.1007/978-3-319-96644-1_8

8.7 Factorial and crossover trial designs are used to increase efficiency.
8.8 The analysis of trial data compares the incidences of disease among treatment groups.

   8.8.1 Measures of effect include relative risk, attributable risk, and number needed to treat.
   8.8.2 The intention-to-treat strategy evaluates all people who were initially randomized and analyzes outcomes according to the original treatment assignments.
   8.8.3 Subgroup analyses assess whether the effects of a treatment differ across subgroups.

8.9 An important potential limitation of randomized trials is restricted external validity due to a relatively healthy study population and a closely monitored study environment.

A randomized trial is a prospective study in humans that evaluates the benefits and harms of an intervention against control procedures.

8.1   Rationale for Randomized Trials

The associations seen in observational studies, including cross-sectional studies, cohort studies, and case-control studies, may or may not indicate a causal impact of the exposure of interest on the disease process. Randomized trials are designed to isolate the causal effects of one or more specific interventions by *assigning* people to different treatments or control procedures.

Randomized studies are applicable only to exposures or treatments that can be administered to people. There is no practical way to assign people to occupational injuries, inherited genetic sequences, recreational drug use, or different levels of air pollution. Moreover, for treatments that can be feasibly dispensed, it may be inappropriate to conduct randomized trials if current knowledge already strongly supports or contradicts the use of the treatment. For example, it would be considered unethical to conduct a randomized trial comparing antimicrobial therapy versus no treatment for acute bloodstream infection, because this condition is life-threatening and antimicrobial therapy is already known to be a highly efficacious treatment. Consequently, randomized trials should be considered when a treatment can be administered in a practical manner *and* when there is ongoing uncertainty regarding the impact of the treatment. The following examples contrast the rationales for conducting randomized trials.

Example 8.1 End-stage kidney disease requires lifelong dialysis or kidney transplantation for survival. Kidney transplantation is more effective than dialysis for removing metabolic waste products and retained fluids. In one observational study, researchers evaluated a group of chronic dialysis patients who were on the kidney transplant waiting list [1]. During the study, some of these patients received a kidney transplant whereas others remained on dialysis. By the end of the study, patients who had received a kidney transplant experienced a 70% lower rate of death compared with those who remained on dialysis.

The hypothesis that kidney transplantation favorably influences survival is supported by the *strong association* (70% lower risk of death) seen in this and other observational studies and *biologic plausibility* for the association based on studies demonstrating superior functional properties of transplantation compared with dialysis. Researchers conducting the study restricted their analyses to patients who were healthy enough to receive a kidney transplant to disentangle the effects of transplantation from potential differences in the health status of transplanted versus non-transplanted individuals. Nonetheless, the best evidence to support the hypothesis that kidney transplantation itself improves survival would come from a randomized trial, in which patients would be *assigned* to either receive a kidney transplant or remain on dialysis. Such a trial would be perceived as unethical, because the totality of existing data already provides compelling evidence for the relative benefits of kidney transplantation.

Example 8.2 Two treatments for myocardial infarction (heart attack) are angioplasty, a procedure to open blocked coronary arteries, and fibrinolysis, a drug that rapidly dissolves blood clots. Patients with myocardial infarction typically receive angioplasty, if they present to a hospital that has the technical capacity to perform this procedure, or fibrinolysis if the hospital is less technically equipped. Observational studies comparing these treatments have reported inconsistent results. The interpretation of these studies is obscured by potential differences in the characteristics of patients who received angioplasty versus those who received fibrinolysis, such as socioeconomic factors and access to centers that perform angioplasty. These characteristics may be difficult to measure reliably. In one randomized trial, investigators recruited more than 1000 patients with acute myocardial infarction who presented to hospitals that lacked the capacity to perform angioplasty [2]. The investigators assigned half of these patients to receive fibrinolysis locally and the other half to immediate transfer to an outside facility for angioplasty. The results of the trial demonstrated a modest relative benefit of angioplasty on the outcome of recurrent myocardial infarction, stroke, or death after 30 days.

This randomized trial was supported by ongoing ambiguity regarding the risks and benefits of angioplasty compared with fibrinolysis and the inability of observational studies to reliably separate the effects of these treatments from the characteristics of patients who received them.

The rationale for performing randomized trials may be appreciated through the concept of *equipoise*, which is defined as the point in which a *rational and informed person has no preference among two or more available treatments*. For example, a rational and informed patient who is receiving chronic dialysis is likely to prefer kidney transplantation over remaining on dialysis based on the totality of observational data and supportive biological evidence. The lack of equipoise for this question impedes a randomized trial on ethical grounds, because it would be considered unethical to *assign* a dialysis patient to remain on dialysis (and withhold kidney transplantation) for the purposes of a trial. In contrast, a rational and informed person would likely have no clear preference between angioplasty and thrombolysis for treating myocardial infarction based on evidence that existed prior to the trial. Equipoise should be viewed as an evolving process that can sometimes by challenged by subsequent research.

Example 8.3 Erythropoietin (EPO) is a hormone produced by the kidneys that stimulates red blood cell production. EPO levels decline in kidney disease, leading anemia (low red cell count). These facts promoted widespread use of EPO treatment in patients with kidney disease in the absence of definitive trials. To challenge the assumption of benefit from EPO, researchers assigned more than 4000 kidney disease patients to receive either EPO treatment or an inert substance packaged to look like EPO (placebo) [3]. Many medical experts and patients believed this trial to be unethical, arguing that a rational and informed person with kidney disease should clearly prefer EPO to a placebo based on existing knowledge. Such concerns slowed trial recruitment; however, the study was eventually completed. Surprisingly, EPO treatment was found to be associated with *greater* risks of stroke and venous thrombosis and had *no impact* on survival. Had the investigators not challenged the assumption of equipoise in this setting, such information would have remained unknown.

8.2   General Design of Randomized Trials

Randomized trials are *prospective studies* that evaluate outcomes that occur over time. The general design is similar to that of cohort studies, described in Chap. 6. The major distinction is that trials *assign* people to one or more interventions or control procedures, whereas cohort studies measure exposures that occur "naturally." For example, the clinical trial of EPO used a random process to assign participants to receive either EPO treatment or a placebo. Randomization was used to dissociate the effects of EPO treatment from the characteristics of patients who received this treatment. In contrast, EPO use in a cohort (observational) study would be influenced by the health characteristics and preferences of the study subjects and the prescribing habits of their physicians.

8.3   Trial Populations

Several considerations inform the selection of the study population in randomized trials, including the definition of the target condition, suspected nonadherence with the study treatment, comorbidity, safety, current use of the study treatment, and the applicability of the trial results.

8.3.1   Definition of the Target Condition

Randomized trials evaluate the impact of treatments among people who have the condition targeted by these treatments. The target condition may be a disease, such as myocardial infarction or cancer. In other instances, trials may target *risk factors* for a disease, such as trials comparing the impact of different smoking cessation strategies on the incidence of myocardial infarction among otherwise healthy smokers.

The findings obtained in randomized trials will have greater applicability if the target condition is defined using pragmatic (practical) methods similar to those used in real-world settings. For example, a trial compared two different surgical procedures for aortic valve replacement among patients with moderate-severe aortic valve stenosis. Researchers conducting this trial defined aortic stenosis by echocardiographic measurements of aortic valve area and patient reported symptoms of the disease. Similar procedures are used to determine the presence and severity of aortic valve disease in clinical practice, facilitating applicability of the trial results to routine healthcare settings. In other instances, the condition targeted by trials may be less readily applicable to clinical care.

Example 8.4 HMG-CoA reductase inhibitors (statins) reduce serum cholesterol levels and decrease the risk of cardiovascular outcomes. Statins also possess anti-inflammatory properties, which may explain some of their benefit. To explore this hypothesis, researchers conducted a randomized trial comparing rosuvastatin to placebo in 17,802 people who had normal serum cholesterol levels but elevated levels of C-reactive protein (CRP), a marker of chronic inflammation [4]. By the end of the study, rosuvastatin treatment was associated with a significant reduction in the incidence of major cardiovascular events.

Restricting the study population to people who had normal serum cholesterol levels, but evidence of chronic inflammation, provides intriguing evidence that anti-inflammatory actions of statins may contribute to their cardioprotective effects. However, the use of an elevated serum CRP level to define entry into the trial restricts applicability of the results, because, at present, CRP levels are infrequently measured in clinical practice. The results of the trial do not address whether rosuvastatin treatment might provide similar benefit to people who have normal cholesterol levels, regardless of their CRP level.

8.3.2   Exclusion of People Suspected to Have Difficulty Adhering to the Study Treatments

Randomized trials typically select people who have a high likelihood of adhering to the study interventions and completing the planned study procedures, because removing participants after randomization jeopardizes the validity of trial results.

One method to improve adherence is called a *run-in period*, in which potential participants receive some form of treatment (or a placebo) *before randomization*. For example, researchers conducting the rosuvastatin trial could first provide all eligible participants with a 1-month supply of placebo capsules and assess compliance by counting the number of capsules remaining at the end of the month. Individuals who are found to be adherent with the run-in procedure would subsequently undergo randomization to either rosuvastatin or a placebo.

8.3.3   Exclusion of People Who Have Comorbid Conditions

Randomizing large numbers of people provides a reasonable degree of confidence that the presence and severity of comorbid conditions will be similar between the treatment and control groups. Consequently, associations seen in large randomized trials are unlikely to be biased by differences in the comorbidity of participants who are assigned to active treatment versus control procedures. Nonetheless, trials often exclude people with serious underlying diseases, such as advanced heart failure or liver disease, as well as people with major physical or psychosocial limitations. Such exclusions are based on several assumptions:

- People with extensive comorbidity are less likely to respond to the study treatments.
- People with extensive comorbidity may incur the trial outcome irrespective of treatment.
- People with extensive comorbidity are less likely to comply with the study procedures.
- People with extensive comorbidity are more likely to experience adverse events.
- People with extensive comorbidity may die before completing the study.

These assumptions are often unproven. Some exclusions for comorbidity can increase the ability of a trial to accurately ascertain the direct benefits and harms of a treatment of interest. However, the overzealous use of exclusions can create unrealistically healthy trial populations that poorly reflect characteristics of "typical" people with the condition targeted by trials.

8.3.4   Exclusion of People Who Are Already Receiving the Study Treatment

For trials of treatments that are already in current use, it may be difficult to recruit people who are naive to treatment. Consider a hypothetical trial to evaluate whether vitamin C supplementation can reduce chronic pain symptoms among patients with fibromyalgia. Recruitment for such a trial may be impeded by the widespread use of multivitamins containing vitamin C. The researchers could ask current multivitamin users to temporarily discontinue this treatment for the purposes of trial participation. After a suitable washout period, eligible participants would then be randomly assigned to either vitamin C treatment or a placebo. Temporary cessation of an existing treatment is justified for trial participation if discontinuation of the treatment can be performed safely and if the effects of the treatment are relatively short-lived.

A previous history of non-response to one of the study treatments could potentially predispose a trial population toward a favorable response to one of the other treatments.

Example 8.5 A randomized trial compared surgical placement of an adjustable gastric band to a very low-calorie diet combined with exercise counseling [5]. The primary outcome of the trial was the amount of weight loss after 2 years. Requirements for trial entry included a body mass index >30 kg/m^2 and previous attempts to lose weight by nonsurgical methods.

The inclusion criteria imply previous failure to adequately lose weight by conventional means, such as diet and exercise. The relative impact of surgery in this trial may be amplified when compared with a treatment that was previously found to be ineffective. The findings from this trial apply specifically to people who have been unable to lose weight without surgery.

8.3.5 Exclusion for Safety

People who have a high likelihood of incurring harm from the study interventions cannot be safely enrolled in a randomized trial. Examples of exclusions for safety include a known allergy or adverse reaction to a study drug or a definitive contraindication to planned surgical procedures. A run-in period can also be used to reduce the possibility of harm in trials.

Example 8.6 Angiotensin-converting enzyme inhibitors and angiotensin receptor blockers (ARBs) are medications used to slow the progression of diabetic kidney disease. A randomized trial compared ARB treatment alone versus the combination of these two treatments for slowing disease progression [6]. A known complication of both medications is an increase in serum potassium levels. To reduce the possibility of this adverse event occurring during the trial, the researchers first administered an ARB to all eligible participants during a run-in period. They carefully monitored for changes in serum potassium levels during this period and excluded people who developed a significant increase with treatment. The remaining participants were then randomly assigned to receive either ARB treatment alone or combination therapy. This strategy reduced, but did not fully eliminate, the occurrence of high potassium levels in the trial.

The applicability of results obtained from trials that include a run-in period is restricted to people who can complete similar procedures. Applicability will be greatest for run-in procedures designed to parallel the strategies used in clinical practice. The run-in period used in the ARB trial above was similar to the approach used in practice, in which clinicians frequently monitor serum potassium levels immediately after starting ARB treatment and stop this treatment if potassium levels become too high.

8.3.6 Broadly Inclusive Healthcare Settings Promote Applicability of Trial Results

Clinical trials have the greatest potential to influence healthcare if they are conducted among diverse groups of people who have the condition under treatment. For example, the trial of EPO (Example 8.3) recruited patients from 623 practice sites in 24 countries. This approach reduced the possibility that unique attributes of patients who received care at a particular clinic or the practice patterns of individual clinics could have disproportionately impacted the results.

8.4 Interventions and Control Procedures

8.4.1 Intervention

The intervention in a randomized trial can be a medication, a procedure, a lifestyle modification, counseling, or any form of therapy that can be feasibly administered in a trial setting. In many instances, previous data are used to guide the intensity and frequency of trial interventions. For example, the dose and duration of medications administered in trials are often informed by the results of previous dose-finding studies. Similarly, details of specific dietary interventions in trials may be selected based on previous observational data and clinical guidelines.

Sometimes the intervention in a trial can be the target of a treatment. For example, a clinical trial tested the risks and benefits of intensive blood pressure reduction by randomly assigning 9361 people to a systolic blood pressure target of either <140 mmHg or <120 mmHg. The researchers were permitted to use different types and dosages of antihypertensive medications to achieve these blood pressure goals. Clinical trials of treatment targets are specifically designed to determine the values and harms of different achieved values of treatments but are not suited to evaluate the effects of the treatments themselves, because such effects are intermixed with the biological response to treatment.

8.4.2 Control Procedures

Randomized trials compare the values and harms of one or more treatments to those of control procedures. Choices of control procedures include the administration of a placebo, a similar treatment, delayed treatment, an accepted standard of care, or no treatment at all. Equipoise helps to inform the control procedures of trials, because it is unethical to assign people to procedures that are known to be inferior to the study treatment.

8.4.2.1 Placebo

A placebo is a substance or procedure that is perceived as therapy but has no biologic or therapeutic activity. Examples of placebos include a pill that appears identical to a study medication but lacks the active ingredient and a skin incision created under sedation to mimic a surgical procedure. Placebos are used in clinical trials to separate the biologic and therapeutic effects of an intervention from the effects of the study procedures and to prevent participants and researchers from knowing the status of the interventions, a process called *blinding*.

Example 8.7 A randomized trial assigned 440 middle-aged men and women with major depression to receive either a new antidepressant medication or an identical-appearing capsule that contained only gelatin (placebo). All participants returned to the study center each week to complete questionnaires regarding depression symptoms and to receive counseling about non-pharmacologic therapies for depression, such as regular exercise. At the end of the study, depression scores improved in 70% of participants who were assigned to the new medication and 50% of participants who were assigned to placebo.

The 50% improvement in depression symptoms seen in the placebo group reflects the combined impact of the study procedures, which included weekly in-person visits, counseling regarding supportive therapies for depression, and the belief that pharmacologic therapy will be effective. The additional improvement in depression symptoms observed in the active treatment groups presumably reflects the biological impact of the new medication itself on these symptoms. The use of a placebo also prevented participants in this study from knowing which treatment they were receiving, minimizing the possibility that such knowledge would influence their responses to the depression questionnaires.

8.4.2.2 Delayed Treatment

Clinical trials can be used to determine the optimal timing of life-saving therapies that cannot be withheld for ethical reasons. For example, it would be unethical to conduct a trial comparing antiretroviral medications to a placebo among patients with advanced HIV disease, because antiretroviral therapy is essential for survival in this setting. However, the risks and benefits of antiretroviral treatment in early HIV disease were less clear.

Example 8.8 A clinical trial recruited 4685 adult HIV patients who had no symptoms of the disease and a CD4 lymphocyte count >500 cells/mm^3. The investigators randomly assigned half of the participants to receive immediate antiretroviral treatment and the other half to a delayed treatment strategy that required the development of an HIV complication or a CD4 count <350 cells/mm^3. Participants who were assigned to delayed treatment began therapy about 3 years later than those assigned to early treatment. The frequency of serious adverse outcomes, including AIDS-related events or death, was 1.8% in the immediate treatment group versus 4.1% in the delayed treatment group [7]. The use of a delayed treatment comparison group provided important new information regarding the treatment of early HIV disease.

8.4.2.3   Pre-existing Standard of Care

A currently accepted standard of care may be a necessary control procedure in trials of serious diseases that require treatment. For example, a clinical trial examined the efficacy of mycophenolate, an immunosuppressant medication, as maintenance therapy for systemic lupus erythematosus, a serious autoimmune disorder. To ensure that all participants received appropriate medical care, the researchers assigned half of the participants to receive mycophenolate and the other half to receive azathioprine, another immunosuppressant medication that was the accepted maintenance therapy for lupus at the time of the trial.

8.4.2.4   No Treatment

Some trials select no treatment as the comparison group to assess the pragmatic, or real-world, risks and benefits of an intervention. Caregivers in clinical practice are faced with decisions regarding whether to prescribe medications, recommend counseling, provide non-pharmacologic treatments, or observe patients over time; placebos are *not* part of routine care. Moreover, in real-world settings, patients who receive no treatment are free to choose among other therapies outside of their medical care.

8.5   Outcomes of Trials

8.5.1   Capture Important Benefits and Harms of the Intervention

Ideally, the outcomes selected in trials should capture the important clinical, biological, and/or societal effects of the study treatments. Consider the clinical trial comparing angioplasty to fibrinolysis for acute myocardial infraction (Example 8.2). Outcomes that assess the relative benefits of these interventions include the resolution of chest pain, recurrent episodes of myocardial infarction, and death due to coronary heart disease. Outcomes that compare the relative safety of these treatments include procedural complications, which can occur with angioplasty, and major bleeding episodes, a known side effect of thrombolysis.

An important consideration for selecting trial outcomes is the ability to measure the outcome with a high degree of certainty. The valid assessment of chest pain and other cardiac symptoms as trial outcomes would require the use of instruments designed to quantify these symptoms in a reproducible manner. The selection of recurrent myocardial infarction as a trial outcome would ideally require validation of these events based on expert review of medical record data obtained throughout the trial.

8.5.2   Types of Outcomes

The outcomes of randomized trials can be *clinical events*, such as stroke, hip fracture, or cancer recurrence, or *quantitative outcomes*, such as the change in tumor size, blood pressure, or viral counts. The ascertainment of outcomes in randomized trials requires prospective follow-up procedures, such as telephone contacts, in-person exams, review of electronic medical records, or linkage with registries. Quantitative outcomes require follow-up study visits to conduct the procedures needed to measure these outcomes, such as imaging studies, blood collection, or tests of physical performance.

8.5.3   Mortality Outcomes

All-cause mortality is often selected as an outcome of clinical trials or is assessed in combination with other trial outcomes. One advantage of evaluating all-cause mortality is that this outcome is relatively easy to determine accurately, whereas specific causes of death may be more difficult to classify. A second advantage is that survival status can often be determined from administrative sources, such as government registries. However, all-cause mortality is influenced by many factors that are unlikely to be related to treatments that target a single disease pathway. The inclusion of all-cause mortality as an outcome, or part of an outcome, in clinical trials may substantially dilute the effects of an intervention and miss important values and harms of that intervention [8]. For example, the trial comparing angioplasty with fibrinolysis found that angioplasty reduced the risk of recurrent myocardial infarction by 33%, whereas the relative benefit of angioplasty on mortality was considerably smaller and not statistically significant. The relatively weak effects of angioplasty on all-cause mortality do not dismiss the important merits of this treatment specifically on cardiovascular outcomes.

8.5.4   Surrogate Outcomes

Randomized trials cannot always assess clinical outcomes, particularly if such outcomes are uncommon or require a long follow-up period for accrual. For example, a trial of a new osteoporosis medication would ideally evaluate the impact of this treatment on fractures, because fracture outcomes capture the presumed biological effects of the treatment and are important to patients and the healthcare system. However, fractures occur infrequently and may require years of follow-up for accrual of sufficient numbers for comparison. A fracture trial may be prohibitively expensive due to sample size and follow-up requirements.

A common approach to this problem is the use of *surrogate endpoints*, which are substitutes for direct measurements of how a patient feels, functions, or survives. An ideal surrogate endpoint is a characteristic that changes in response to treatment in a manner that is consistent with the clinical benefits and harms of that treatment. For example, bone mineral density is considered to be a valid surrogate endpoint for fracture, because osteoporosis treatments improve bone mineral density in a manner that corresponds with their protective effects on fracture. The use of bone mineral density as a surrogate endpoint for fracture reduces the cost and complexity of osteoporosis trials, creating opportunities for studying new potential therapies for this disease. On the other hand, some outcomes used as surrogates have been found wanting.

Example 8.9 Encainide, flecainide, and moricizine are medications designed to suppress cardiac arrhythmias. In preliminary studies, these drugs reduced the frequency of premature ventricular contractions (PVCs), an early indicator of some types of cardiac arrhythmias. In the Cardiac Arrhythmia Suppression Trial (CAST), investigators assigned 1727 patients with asymptomatic cardiac arrhythmias to one of these medications or a placebo [9]. The drugs effectively suppressed PVCs during the trial but substantially *increased* the risk of death due to cardiac arrhythmia and other cardiovascular causes, prompting early termination of the trial.

The assertion that PVCs were a surrogate endpoint for lethal cardiac arrhythmias was based on observational data reporting associations of PVCs with cardiac death. Such associations are insufficient for demonstrating that PVCs are a surrogate endpoint for lethal arrhythmia. The trial found that PVCs did *not* change in response to treatment in a manner that corresponded with the clinical benefits or harms of treatment. In fact, these treatments had opposing effects on PVCs and cardiac death.

8.5.5   Premature Termination of Trials

An independent data safety and monitoring board (DSMB) is usually required to monitor the progress of trials and ensure the safety of participants. The DSMB, which should include clinical experts and statisticians, conducts scheduled meetings to review accruing unblinded trial data. The DSMB can elect to terminate a trial prematurely in the event of overwhelming evidence of benefit, concerns regarding safety, or projected futility.

8.6   Procedures to Promote Internal Validity of Trials

Clinical trials use *randomization, blinding,* and *concealment* to promote internal validity, which describes the ability of a trial to accurately determine the benefits and harms of the study treatments within the selected trial population and monitoring environment.

8.6.1   Randomization

Randomization is used to balance the characteristics of trial participants – both measured and unmeasured – across the treatment groups to assess the causal impact of one or more treatments of interest. Table 8.1 presents baseline characteristics from two hypothetical randomized trials that assign 100 or 1000 people with chronic migraine headache to either a new headache medication or no treatment at all.

The smaller trial achieves reasonable similarity in mean age and the proportion of female participants across the treatment groups. However, the frequency of previous stroke is dissimilar. Larger numbers of randomized participants are needed to achieve balance in uncommon characteristics, such as previous stroke.

Dissimilarities in participant characteristics across treatment groups in randomized trials are likely to represent chance occurrences. The contrasting proportions of previous stroke and the smaller imbalances in age and sex seen in the 100-person migraine trial likely occurred due to chance and can be addressed by randomizing larger numbers of participants. In contrast, potential imbalances in participant characteristics seen in observational studies may reflect systematic differences that cannot be addressed by increasing the size of a study. For example, consider a hypothetical observational study comparing the new migraine medication with no treatment among people with chronic headache. The characteristics of people who receive the new medication may differ from those who do not receive this medication

Table 8.1   Characteristics of trial participants as a function of sample size

	Trial 1		Trial 2	
	Study drug	No treatment	Study drug	No treatment
Number of participants	50	50	500	500
Mean age (years)	49.5	48.7	49.1	49.0
Female (%)	63.2	69.1	65.8	66.2
Previous stroke (%)	4.0	0	3.2	2.7

based on the *reasons* for its use, such as the severity of headache symptoms or the type of health insurance coverage. Such sytematic differences are not addressed by increasing the sample size.

Simple randomization procedures are those that perform randomization without regard to previous treatment assignments. A coin flip is an example of simple randomization. Such procedures work well in larger trials but may generate unequally sized treatment groups and leave residual imbalance in specific characteristics in smaller trials. For example, the use of a coin flip to assign 100 people to either the new migraine headache medication or no treatment may not allocate exactly 50 people to each group.

Restricted randomization strategies are more complex procedures used to increase the degree of similarity across treatment and control groups in trials. These procedures must be planned prior to implementation of a trial and incorporated into the randomization process. *Block randomization* is a restricted randomization strategy that performs randomization within smaller groups of participants. A sample block randomization strategy for the 100-person migraine medication trial would be to create 10 bins, each containing 10 slips of paper. Within each bin, five slips would indicate the study medication, and five would indicate no treatment. The first ten enrolled participants would randomly select a slip of paper from the first bin, ensuring that exactly five people are assigned to each treatment group within that bin. This procedure would then be repeated over successive bins (blocks). Block randomization is particularly helpful for ensuring similarly sized treatment groups in the event of premature termination of a trial.

To prevent chance imbalances in specific characteristics from undermining the validity of smaller trials, a similar procedure called stratified randomization can be used to create similarity in one or more pre-specified characteristics across treatment groups. For example, the 100-person headache medication trial could create one bin containing 10 slips of paper for participants with a previous history of stroke and another bin containing 90 slips of paper for participants without a stroke history. Within each bin, exactly half of the slips would indicate study medication and the other half would indicate no treatment. Enrolled participants would select a slip of paper from the bin corresponding to their previous stroke history, ensuring equal proportions of previous stroke across the treatment and control groups. This procedure can be useful for creating similarity in one or a small number of disease risk factors in smaller trials but will increase complexity of the trial.

8.6.2 Blinding

Participant awareness of which treatment they are receiving may influence their responses to the trial procedures and impact their behaviors outside of the trial. For example, participants in the migraine medication trial received either the new medication or no treatment at all, allowing them to recognize which treatment they were receiving. Such knowledge may influence their reporting of headache symptoms, a subjectively measured outcome, and could differentially impact their use of other headache therapies on their own. Bias may also occur if investigators are aware of the treatment assignments, because such knowledge could influence their analyses.

Blinding describes study procedures used to prevent participants and investigators from knowing the identity of the interventions received throughout the duration of a trial. A *single blind* study describes blinding of only the participants. A *double-blind* study describes blinding of both the participants and the investigators. Blinding is performed by the use of control treatments that are indistinguishable from the study treatments (placebo). In some instances, it may not be possible to blind participants to the identity of the study treatments, such as in trials of exercise programs, counseling, or invasive surgical procedures. In such instances, the potential problem of differential outcome reporting can be mitigated by the use of objectively measured trial outcomes, if such outcomes are appropriate.

8.6.3   Concealment of Treatment Allocation

The random process used to allocate treatments in trials can be jeopardized if the personnel who administer these treatments are aware of the planned assignments. For example, suppose that the migraine medication trial planned to use a placebo, instead of no treatment, and proposed to assign participants to either the new medication or placebo within randomized blocks of four. Allocation of the first three treatments within a block would necessarily reveal the identity of the fourth treatment and could consciously or subconsciously influence study personnel to guide participants toward a specific treatment group, such as steering participants who have more severe headache symptoms toward active treatment. Concealment of treatment allocation is accomplished by the use of a third party, such as an investigational pharmacy, to perform the randomization and allocate the study treatments but withhold such information from study personnel, investigators, and participants until the end of the study.

8.6.4   Efficacy and Effectiveness

Efficacy refers to the direct benefits and harms of an intervention observed under idealized conditions. Trials that seek to determine efficacy tend to employ stringent inclusion criteria, utilize detailed procedures to measure trial outcomes with a high degree of accuracy, and closely monitor participants to encourage compliance and ensure safety. *Effectiveness* refers to the practical impact of an intervention among diverse groups of people in realistic settings. Trials that favor effectiveness tend to recruit people from communities and general healthcare settings, apply relatively few exclusion criteria, and employ practical monitoring procedures that can be readily duplicated in real-world settings. Efficacy and effectiveness are descriptive terms used to characterize opposing strategies of trial design. Few trials would be characterized as exclusively one of these types. Most trials attempt to balance attributes of efficacy and effectiveness based on the study question of interest.

8.6.5 Trial Reporting

The results of randomized trials tend to have a disproportionate influence on clinical care. Consequently, mechanisms have been established to promote transparency surrounding the design, conduct, analysis, and reporting of trials. ClinicalTrials.gov (https://clinicaltrials.gov) is a registry of publicly and privately supported trials conducted around the world. Researchers are encouraged to publish details of their planned research in this registry *before implementation of a trial*. The registry process is intended to minimize biases due to data-driven changes in the analysis of trials and reduce publication bias, in which negative results are withheld.

The CONSORT (Consolidated Standards of Reporting Trials) guidelines are a checklist of standardized items used to facilitate the reporting of trial results and simplify their interpretation (http://www.consort-statement.org). CONSORT guidelines include recommended procedures for the reporting of trial populations, recruitment methods, exclusion criteria, randomization, blinding, analysis, funding, and other key aspects of clinical trials.

8.7 Specific Trial Designs

8.7.1 Factorial Trials

In some instances, researchers may wish to evaluate more than one treatment within the same trial. For example, vitamin D and omega-3 fatty acids are dietary supplements that possess broad antiproliferative and anti-inflammatory properties and may prevent the development of certain chronic diseases. Ongoing clinical trials are testing whether these treatments can reduce the incidence of cancer, cardiovascular disease, and fractures. The conventional strategy for evaluating both vitamin D and omega-3 fatty acid treatments would be to assign people to one of three different treatment groups: vitamin D, omega-3 fatty acids, or placebo. This approach is called a *parallel group design*. An alternative strategy would be to create *four* different intervention groups corresponding to each possible combination of treatment and placebo, shown in Table 8.2.

Table 8.2 Factorial design clinical trial of vitamin D and omega-3 fatty acids

	Omega-3 fatty acids	Placebo
Vitamin D	a	b
Placebo	c	d

The above strategy is called a *factorial design trial*. Participants in such a trial would receive *two* identical appearing study medications consisting of either (a) vitamin D plus omega-3 fatty acids, (b) vitamin D plus placebo, (c) omega-3 fatty acids plus placebo, or (d) two placebos. The impact of vitamin D treatment on the study outcomes would then be determined by comparing all participants who receive vitamin D (groups a and b) to all participants who do not receive vitamin D (groups c and d). Analogously, the effects of omega-3 fatty acid treatment would be determined by comparing all participants who receive omega-3 fatty acids (groups a and c) to all participants who do not receive this treatment (groups b and d).

The primary advantage of the factorial design is increased efficiency gained from "borrowing" participants across the treatment groups. Suppose a factorial design trial assigns 3000 people to one of the four treatments groups described in Table 8.2 (750 people in each group). This strategy would compare 1500 people assigned to vitamin D with 1500 people assigned to placebo *and* would compare 1500 people assigned to omega-3 fatty acids with 1500 people assigned to placebo. An identically sized parallel group design trial would compare only 1000 people assigned to vitamin D and 1000 people assigned to omega-3 fatty acids with 1000 people assigned to placebo, reducing the power of the study.

However, the efficiency gained from the factorial design hinges on the assumption that the effect of the interventions on trial outcomes is independent of one another. If the study treatments are found to act synergistically or antagonistically, then combining participants across the treatment groups is no longer valid. For example, if the combination of vitamin D plus omega-3 fatty acid treatment is found to reduce cancer incidence to a much greater degree than the individual effects of each of these treatments, then analyses of vitamin D must be restricted to comparison of vitamin D alone (group b) versus placebo alone (group d), and analyses of omega-3 fatty acids must be restricted to comparison of omega-3 fatty acids alone (group c) versus placebo alone (group d). The presence of interactive effects renders the factorial design *less efficient* than the corresponding parallel group design. A second drawback of factorial design trials is potential difficulty in monitoring adherence with more than one study treatment.

8.7.2 Crossover Trials

For the evaluation of interventions believed to have a rapid impact, another method used to increase the efficiency of trials is a *crossover design*, in which participants receive more than one treatment during the same trial.

Example 8.10 A hypothetical trial compares the impact of two different sodium diets on blood pressure. The researchers randomly assign 40 healthy participants to receive either 2 weeks of a low-sodium diet followed by 2 weeks of a regular sodium diet or the same treatments in reverse order. A research center prepares all meals and snacks during the study to control the amount of sodium intake, and participants are instructed to refrain from consuming other foods or beverages outside of the trial. The study design is depicted in Fig. 8.1.

For the 20 participants who receive the low-sodium diet first, the effect of this diet is determined by the difference in blood pressures between time points A and B. For participants who receive the regular sodium diet first, the effect of the low-sodium diet is calculated as the difference in blood pressures between time points C and D, shown in Table 8.3.

Analogous to factorial design trials, a major advantage of the crossover design is increased efficiency. If all 40 participants complete the trial, then the crossover design will generate 40 low-sodium diet periods for comparison with 40 regular sodium diet periods. A parallel group design trial that randomizes 40 people to either a low-sodium diet or a regular sodium diet would yield only 20 such comparisons. Crossover trials have a second advantage of comparing treatment effects within the same person, eliminating the potential for bias that may arise from chance imbalances in characteristics across treatment groups.

An important requirement for crossover trials is that the study interventions be provided in random order. Figure 8.2 demonstrates the seemingly innocuous strategy of consistently assigning participants to the low-sodium diet first followed by the regular sodium diet.

Non-randomized provision of the treatments creates susceptibility to bias if the other study procedures impact the outcomes under study. In this example, provision of meals prepared by a research center and close monitoring of blood pressures in a trial setting could themselves reduce blood pressure independently of the effects of the sodium diets. Trial procedures tend to have the largest impact at the beginning of a study and dissipate thereafter. Consistently providing the low-sodium diet first would conflate the impact of this diet on blood pressure with that of the other study procedures. Randomizing the order of the treatments is needed to avoid this potential problem.

In most instances, crossover trials require a *washout period* to separate the effects of the study treatments. The appropriate duration of washout can be estimated from the predicted duration of the treatment effects based on other studies. Yet, the biological effects of many treatments may persist after the treatment is no longer detectable, creating uncertainty regarding the optimal duration of washout.

Crossover trials assign participants to more than one treatment within the same trial, prolonging the duration of the trial and increasing the possibility of dropout. Dropout is particularly problematic in crossover trials, because participants serve as their own controls. Withdrawal of participants in crossover studies typically leads to the loss of all study data for those participants, even if they completed some of the study procedures before dropping out.

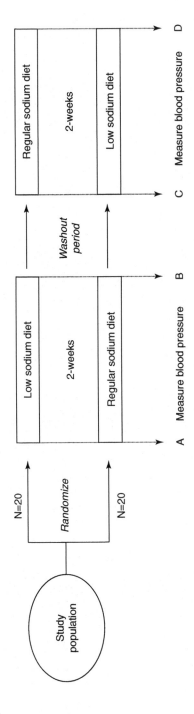

Fig. 8.1 Randomized crossover trial design

Table 8.3 Crossover trial of dietary sodium intake and blood pressure

| Intervention | Effects of the diets on blood pressure | | |
	Effect of regular sodium diet	Effect of low-sodium diet	Comparison of diet effects
Low-sodium diet first	D-C	B-A	(D-C) – (B-A)
Regular sodium diet first	B-A	D-C	(B-A) – (D-C)

8.7.3   Phases of Drug Development

Human drug development proceeds through an organized series of *phases*. Phase I and II studies may not be randomized trials but are used to develop randomized phase III studies.

8.7.3.1   Phase I Studies

Phase I studies are designed to understand how well a new drug is tolerated in a small number of people. Participants in phase I studies are usually healthy volunteers but may also be people who have the disease targeted by the new drug. Phase I studies administer escalating dosages of an experimental drug under carefully supervised conditions to determine pharmacokinetics and maximal tolerable dosages. The data from phase I studies are used to inform dosing in phase II studies.

8.7.3.2   Phase II Studies

Phase II studies are designed to assess the biologic activity of a new drug. These studies administer tolerable dosages, determined from phase I studies, to people who have the disease or condition targeted by the drug. The outcomes of phase II studies are *biologic markers* and *surrogate endpoints*, such as the change in tumor size or the reduction in viral counts, rather than clinical events. The results of phase II studies are used to inform phase III studies.

8.7.3.3   Phase III Studies

Phase III studies are *randomized clinical trials* designed to determine the impact of a new drug on *clinically relevant outcomes*. Compared to phase II studies, phase III studies are conducted among larger groups of participants, include a longer duration of follow-up, and evaluate clinical outcomes, such as fracture, stroke, or cancer survival. Regulatory approval for new drugs is based on successful results from one or more phase III studies.

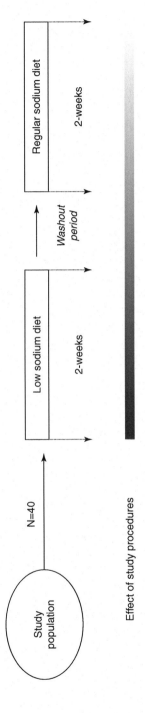

Fig. 8.2 Crossover study with non-randomized treatment order

8.7.3.4 Phase IV Studies

"Phase IV" is a broad term used to describe studies of drug *effectiveness* typically conducted after regulatory approval. These studies assess the real-world values and harms of drugs in more realistic settings than those of phase III studies, which tend to recruit relatively healthier people who have the condition targeted by the treatment and monitor safety under controlled conditions. Stated another way, phase II and III studies tend to focus on drug efficacy, whereas phase IV studies tend to focus on drug effectiveness. Phase IV studies can assume a variety of designs, including meta-analyses, observational studies, and randomized trials. These studies are important for identifying uncommon effects of drugs that may be missed in phase III studies.

Example 8.11 Rofecoxib, a selective inhibitor of the cyclooxygenase-2 enzyme, was developed to relieve musculoskeletal pain while exhibiting fewer gastrointestinal side effects than traditional nonsteroidal anti-inflammatory drugs (NSAIDs). In phase III trials, patients who received rofecoxib experienced modestly higher rates of cardiovascular events compared with those who received NSAIDs; however, the number of these outcomes was small, and mechanisms to explain this finding were initially lacking. Following regulatory approval of rofecoxib, an analysis combined the results of several randomized trials to demonstrate a clear relationship between rofecoxib treatment and a greater incidence of cardiovascular outcomes. The presumed mechanism to explain these adverse effects is selective inhibition of prostacyclin synthesis by rofecoxib, thereby promoting thrombosis. Based on these data and similar findings from other post-marketing trials, rofecoxib was subsequently withdrawn from the market.

8.8 Analysis of Clinical Trial Data

8.8.1 Measures of Effect

The analysis of randomized trial data is conceptually similar to the strategy used for cohort studies. The first step is to calculate the *incidence* (proportions or rates) of the study outcome in each treatment group. The second step is to compare the incidences among the treatment groups using relative risk or other measure of effect. Consider data from the randomized trial comparing rosuvastatin to placebo (Example 8.4). The primary outcome was the development of a major cardiovascular event, defined as myocardial infarction, angina, stroke, or cardiovascular death, over a median of 1.9 years of follow-up, shown in Table 8.4.

Table 8.4 Cardiovascular outcomes in the randomized trial of rosuvastatin

	Number of participants	Number of outcomes	Cumulative incidence (per 100 people)	Incidence rate per 100 person-years
Rosuvastatin	8901	142	1.60	0.77
Placebo	8901	251	2.82	1.36

8.8.1.1 Relative Risk

Relative risk is ideally calculated using incidence rates to account for person time:

$$\text{Relative risk} = \frac{\text{Incidence(treated)}}{\text{Incidence(untreated)}} = \frac{0.77\,\text{events per 100 person} - \text{years}}{1.36\,\text{events per 100 person} - \text{years}}$$
$$= 0.57\,(\text{no units})$$

This relative risk can be interpreted as, "rosuvastatin treatment is associated with a 43% lower incidence of the composite cardiovascular outcome compared with placebo." The "43% lower" derives from the fact that 0.57 is 43% lower than 1.0, which denotes the relative risk that would be observed if rosuvastatin had no impact on the outcome. The large number of randomized participants provides reassurance that this observed difference in cardiovascular outcomes is likely due to rosuvastatin treatment itself. Therefore, the relative risk may also be interpreted as, "rosuvastatin *reduces* the risk of the compsite cardiovascular outcome by 43% compared with placebo."

8.8.1.2 Attributable Risk

The attributable risk can also be calculated from the incidence rate data:

$$\text{Attributable risk} = \text{Incidence(untreated)} - \text{Incidence(treated)}$$
$$= 1.36\,\text{events per 100 person} - \text{years} - 0.77\,\text{events per 100 person} - \text{years}$$
$$= 0.59\,\text{events per 100 person} - \text{years}$$

Attributable risk describes the impact of an intervention on a population. As depicted in Fig. 8.3, there were an additional 0.59 cardiovascular outcomes per 100 person-years in the placebo group of the rosuvastatin trial. The large randomized design provides a reasonable degree of certainty that these extra events were due to the lack of rosuvastatin treatment. Stated another way, an additional 0.59 cardiovascular

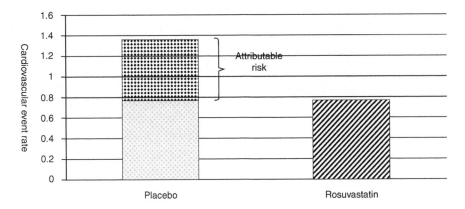

Fig. 8.3 Attributable risk of cardiovascular events associated with rosuvastatin treatment

events per 100 person-years could potentially be prevented by treating people similar to those in the placebo group with rosuvastatin.

Attributable risk provides important complementary information to the relative risk. The 43% relative reduction in the composite outcome associated with rosuvastatin treatment masks the very low rates of this outcome in either treatment group; most participants in this trial did not experience a cardiovascular event whether they were assigned to rosuvastatin or placebo. Such information is important for deciding whether to initiate rosuvastatin treatment.

8.8.1.3 Number Needed to Treat or Harm

The attributable risk can also be used to estimate the number of people who would need to be treated with an intervention to cause or prevent a single instance of an outcome.

$$\text{Number needed to treat or harm} = \frac{1}{\text{Absolute value}\left(\text{attributable risk}\right)}$$

For ease of interpretation, calculation of the number needed to treat will be presented using attributable risks derived from the cumulative incidences rather than the incidence rates.

$$\text{Attributable risk} = \text{Incidence}\left(\text{untreated}\right) - \text{Incidence}\left(\text{treated}\right)$$

Based on the incidence proportion data in Table 8.4:

$$\text{Attributable risk} = \frac{2.82\,\text{events}}{100\,\text{people}} - \frac{1.60\,\text{events}}{100\,\text{people}} = \frac{1.22\,\text{events}}{100\,\text{people}}\left(\text{over}\,1.9\,\text{years follow} - \text{up}\right)$$

The number of people who would need to be treated with rosuvastatin to prevent a single episode of the composite cardiovascular outcome would be calculated as:

$$\text{Number needed to treat} = \frac{1}{\text{abs}\left(1.22\,\text{events}\,/\,100\,\text{people}\right)} = \frac{100\,\text{people}}{1.22\,\text{events}} = \frac{82\,\text{people}}{\text{Event}}$$

Treating 82 people who are like those in the trial with rosuvastatin would be expected to prevent one cardiovascular event. A similar calculation can be performed for harm using the adverse event data from trials. For example, the cumulative incidence of diabetes, a potential side effect of statin therapy, was 3.0% in the rosuvastatin group and 2.4% in the placebo group.

$$\text{Attributable risk} = \text{Incidence}\left(\text{untreated}\right) - \text{Incidence}\left(\text{treated}\right)$$
$$= \frac{2.4\,\text{events}}{100\,\text{people}} - \frac{3.0\,\text{events}}{100\,\text{people}} = \frac{-0.6\,\text{events}}{100\,\text{people}}$$

$$\text{Number needed to harm} = \frac{1}{\left(0.6\,\text{events per}\,100\,\text{people}\right)} = \frac{167\,\text{people}}{\text{Event}}$$

Treatment of every 167 people with rosuvastatin, instead of a placebo, would be expected to cause one additional case of diabetes.

8.8.1.4 Changes in Quantitative Outcomes

Some randomized trials, such as phase II studies, assess quantitative characteristics, such as the change in myocardial infarct size, asthma symptoms, or platelet counts. A simple analytic approach for these types of data is to calculate the change from beginning to end of the trial. For example, the clinical trial comparing laparoscopic band surgery to a very low-calorie diet plus counseling (Example 8.5) evaluated the impact of these treatments on the amount of weight loss after 24 months.

	Participants	Initial weight	Final weight (24 months)	Change
Lap band surgery	40	95.0 kg	74.5 kg	20.5 kg
Diet	40	94.8 kg	89.5 kg	5.3 kg

Difference in weight change = 20.5 kg − 5.3 kg = 15.2 kg

For quantitative outcomes obtained at multiple time points during a trial, more complex statistical methods are typically used to compare slopes or other measures of trajectory over time.

8.8.2 Intention-To-Treat Analysis

Randomized trials assign participants to interventions at the beginning of the trial. However, some participants may discontinue treatment or change treatments after the trial is underway. For example, in the rosuvastatin trial, some people initially assigned to rosuvastatin treatment may stop taking this medication during the trial, possibly due to intolerable side effects. How should outcomes be counted among participants who incur the outcome *after* stopping or switching treatment?

One analytic strategy would be to ignore outcomes that occur after discontinuation of the study treatments. This approach would exclude cardiovascular events that transpired after stopping rosuvastatin in attempt to reflect the participants' "actual" treatment status at the time they experienced the outcome. However, treatment discontinuation may be more likely to occur in the rosuvastatin group and participants who discontinue treatment may be atypical in their likelihood of developing the outcome under investigation.

A second strategy would be to assign outcomes that occur after stopping treatment to the placebo group. The approach presumes that stopping rosuvastatin is analogous to switching to an inert placebo. However, if relatively sicker participants were to preferentially discontinue rosuvastatin treatment during the trial, then this strategy will also be susceptible to bias.

The first two procedures, which are often called "per-protocol" or "as-treated" analyses, disrupt the initial balance in participant characteristics created by randomization. The use of such analyses creates uncertainty as to whether the observed impact of treatments may be distorted by the health status of participants who stop or switch treatments during the trial. Although there may be certain instances in which per-protocol analyses may be used, special care is required for describing these results and ensuring that bias has not occurred.

A third analytic strategy is to continue to count outcomes that occur after stopping or switching treatments according to the initial treatment assignment. Under such an approach, cardiovascular outcomes that occur after stopping rosuvastatin among participants initially assigned to this treatment would be ascribed to the rosuvastatin group. This strategy is called an *intention-to-treat* analysis and is the only method capable of preserving the original similarity in participant characteristics created by randomization. An intention-to-treat analysis is defined by the *inclusion of all participants who are initially randomized and attribution of all study outcomes to the initial treatment assignments.*

Consider the impact of rosuvastatin discontinuation under an intention-to-treat analysis. As participants assigned to rosuvastatin discontinue this treatment during the trial, the "rosuvastatin" group will become progressively diluted with participants who are no longer taking this medication. Consequently, the cardiovascular outcome rate of this mixed group of rosuvastatin users and nonusers will become more like that of the placebo group, yielding a relative risk that is closer to 1.0 compared to that obtained under perfect adherence. This form of predictable bias is called *bias toward the null.* Under an intention-to-treat analysis, greater discontinuation or switching of the study treatments will typically produce more attenuation of the observed relative risk. The intention-to-treat analysis may report weaker effects of study treatments or falsely report no effect of these treatments, but will generally not exaggerate the effects of treatments. For this reason, bias toward the null is also called "conservative error."

It is important to note that discontinuation or switching of treatments after a trial is underway can lead to bias *under any analytic strategy.* For this reason, clinical trials attempt to select participants who are most likely to adhere to the study treatments throughout the trial and employ procedures to encourage compliance.

Nonetheless, among the available choices, the intention-to-treat approach most closely maintains the initial similarity in characteristics created by randomization and generates a predictable form of bias.

Intention-to-treat analyses may be challenging to perform in trials that evaluate the change in quantitative outcomes. For example, the trial of laparoscopic band surgery evaluated the outcome of weight loss after 2 years, which requires end-of-study weight data. Excluding participants who did not return for follow-up weight measurements would *not* satisfy the requirements of an intention-to-treat analysis, because some of the initially randomized participants would not be included. Methods such as last value carried forward or multiple imputations can be applied to such situations to permit analyses of all people who were initially randomized.

8.8.3 Subgroup Analyses

Typically, randomized trials report the average effect of treatments among all trial participants. *Subgroup analyses* are used to explore whether study treatments may have different benefits and harms among smaller groups of people within a trial population. Subgroup analyses have the potential to identify characteristics that may be associated with particularly strong or weak effects of a treatment. However, subgroup analyses require caution in their interpretation due to the potential for discovering chance differences in treatment effects.

Consider the summary relative risk observed in the rosuvastatin trial: rosuvastatin treatment was associated with a 43% lower relative risk of the composite cardiovascular outcome among all 17,802 participants in the trial. It is possible that rosuvastatin treatment has an even greater impact on cardiovascular endpoints in certain groups of participants. For example, many inherited forms of coronary heart disease cause defects in lipid metabolism, some of which are targeted by rosuvastatin. Could the cardiovascular benefits of rosuvastatin treatment be particularly great among people who have a family history of coronary heart disease? Table 8.5 presents the randomized trial data stratified by a family history of coronary disease.

Table 8.5 Effects of rosuvastatin stratified by a family history of coronary heart disease

	Number of participants	Number of outcomes	Incidence rate per 100 person-years
Family history positive			
Rosuvastatin	997	18	0.91
Placebo	1048	53	2.44
			Relative risk = 0.37
Family history negative			
Rosuvastatin	7904	123	0.75
Placebo	7853	199	1.22
			Relative risk = 0.61

Rosuvastatin reduced the relative incidence of the cardiovascular endpoint by (1.0–0.37) = 63% among participants with a family history of coronary disease but only by (1.0–0.61) = 39% among those without a family history. These subgroup findings suggest that, on the relative risk scale, rosuvastatin treatment may be more cardioprotective among people who have a family history. However, the differential size of treatment effects seen in subgroup analyses must be considered in context with the possibility of chance variation in treatment effects. Several criteria can be used to judge whether the observed difference in the impact of a treatment across subgroups is likely to represent a true differential impact of the treatment on disease:

1. The amount of difference in treatment effects across subgroups is large.
2. The subgroups contain sufficient numbers of people and outcomes for comparison.
3. The differential treatment effects are plausible based on evidence from other studies.
4. The differential treatment effects are replicated in other studies.

For the subgroup analyses in Table 8.5, there is a moderate difference in the size of the effect of rosuvastatin treatment: a 63% reduction in cardiovascular events among people with a family history compared with a 39% reduction among those without a family history. The subgroups contained a reasonably large number of participants; however, the number of cardiovascular outcomes in the family history subgroup was only modest. Biologic plausibility for the observed difference in treatment effects is equivocal. On one hand, rosuvastatin treatment reduces levels of low-density lipoprotein cholesterol (LDL-C) and other components of dyslipidemia that may accompany inherited forms of coronary heart disease. On the other hand, statins prevent cardiovascular outcomes across a wide range of LDL-C levels, including those considered to be in the "normal range." Based on the criteria for evaluating differences in treatment effects, it would be premature to conclude that, among people with a family history of coronary heart disease, rosuvastatin treatment is particularly beneficial for preventing cardiovascular outcomes. Further evidence from other trials is needed to address the possibility of differential effects of statin treatment by family history.

Randomized trials often report subgroup analyses using a *forest plot*. Figure 8.4 presents the forest plot from the rosuvastatin trial.

The squares in the figure represent the relative risk of the composite cardiovascular outcome comparing rosuvastatin treatment with placebo within each subgroup. The size of the squares corresponds with the number of participants and the number of outcomes in the subgroup, and the dashed vertical line indicates the summary relative risk obtained in the full study population.

The horizontal lines represent *95% confidence intervals*. In brief, these intervals estimate the amount of variation in the size of associations that are expected from chance. For example, among people with a family history of coronary disease, the relative risk comparing rosuvastatin to placebo could be as low as 0.15 or as high as 0.60 in the underlying population of similar individuals. *Overlapping confidence intervals within subgroups* suggest that the differential size of the association

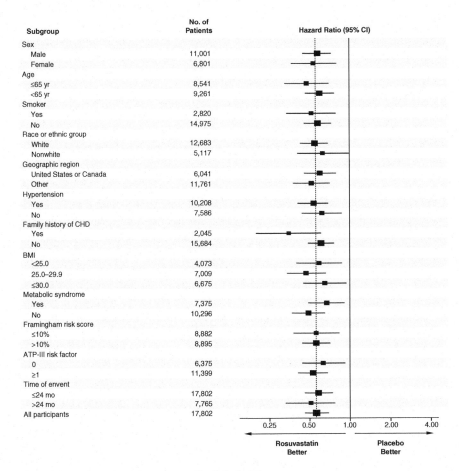

Fig. 8.4 Forest plot from the rosuvastatin clinical trial

observed in the study does *not* exceed that expected from chance. The 95% confidence intervals for people with and without a family history indicate a wide range of possible relative risks for these subgroups, and the overlap of these confidence intervals suggests that the difference in relative risks observed in the trial does *not* exceed chance.

Importantly, observing confidence intervals that overlap with 1.0 in specific subgroups should not be used as evidence that a treatment is ineffective among such people. A common, but mistaken interpretation of the forest plot data would conclude that rosuvastatin treatment reduces cardiovascular outcomes only in whites, but not nonwhites, because the 95% confidence interval for nonwhites overlaps with 1.0. However, relative risks are expected to vary in size across subgroups due to chance. The correct interpretation of the subgroup findings for race is that rosuvastatin treatment reduces the risk of cardiovascular outcomes in the full trial population, including whites and nonwhites, and that the subgroup analyses cannot distinguish whether rosuvastatin treatment has a differential impact on cardiovascular outcomes by race. These contrasting interpretations have important implications for deciding which patients should be treated with rosuvastatin.

8.9 Limitations of Randomized Trials

8.9.1 Limited External Validity (Applicability) of the Trial Population

Randomized trials tend to enroll relatively healthy participants who have a high likelihood of adhering to the study treatments and tolerating these treatments over the duration of the trial. Consequently, the values and harms of treatments observed in randomized trials may differ from those in more general healthcare settings, which include people with a broad range of comorbid illnesses and impairments. Details of participant recruitment reported in trials are useful for appraising the external validity of the trial population. A small proportion of enrolled participants relative to a large number of people screened for a trial suggests lower external validity, indicating caution in applying the trial results to real-world populations.

8.9.2 Limited External Validity (Applicability) of the Trial Environment

Randomized trials are often conducted under controlled conditions to ensure that the study hypothesis is tested in a reproducible and safe fashion. The risks and benefits of treatments observed within the specialized monitoring environments of trials may differ dramatically from those found in clinical practice [10].

Example 8.12 A randomized trial evaluated whether Aldactone, a potassium-sparing diuretic, can reduce the risks of death and hospitalizations in patients with systolic heart failure [11]. The trial assigned 1663 heart failure patients to receive either Aldactone treatment or a placebo. An important safety measure in the trial was elevated serum potassium levels (hyperkalemia), which is a known side effect of Aldactone. Potassium levels were measured monthly during the first 3 months of the trial and then every 3 months thereafter. The risk of serious hyperkalemia was found to be similar between the Aldactone and placebo groups.

Example 8.13 A community-based study of hyperkalemia identified case patients, who had severely elevated serum potassium levels requiring hospitalization, and control patients who did not have this condition from the same community [12]. After adjustment, the use of a potassium-sparing diuretic, including Aldactone, was associated with an approximately 20 times higher risk of serious hyperkalemia compared with no such use.

To summarize, Aldactone treatment had no impact on the incidence of serious hyperkalemia in the randomized trial but was associated with a substantially greater risk of serious hyperkalemia in the observational study. A first consideration is the possibility that the trial participants were healthier than those in the observational study. However, participants in the Aldactone trial had advanced heart failure and were taking multiple heart failure medications. Another possibility is that unmeasured differences in the characteristics of case and control individuals in the observational study distorted the association between Aldactone treatment and hyperkalemia.

However, the most likely source of the discrepancy is the difference in the study environments. The randomized trial frequently monitored serum potassium levels to maximize safety. Even a small increase in potassium levels triggered a reduction in the dose of Aldactone or temporary discontinuation of this treatment. Such intensive monitoring procedures essentially eliminated the risk of serious hyperkalemia in the randomized trial. In contrast, monitoring procedures are far less stringent in clinical practice. The likely conclusion is that both study results are correct. Aldactone does not increase the risk of serious hyperkalemia in the environment of a randomized trial, but strongly increases the risk of this outcome in clinical practice.

8.9.3   Narrow Study Question

Randomized trials are designed to definitively answer a specific focused question by isolating the effects of one or a small number of treatments. Trials are generally not designed to simultaneously test the mechanisms by which these treatments may produce clinical benefits or harms. The results of the Aldactone trial provided a strong rationale for prescribing this medication to patients with systolic heart failure. Other studies are needed to understand *why* Aldactone might produce such a large survival benefit. Moreover, randomized trials are generally not ideal for exploring the effects of many different treatments, dosages, or combinations of treatments, as this would notably dilute the size of each intervention group.

8.9.4   Randomized Design Accounts Only for Confounding

Randomized trials are designed to increase the degree of similarity in participant characteristics across the treatment groups to minimize confounding as a potential study flaw. Freedom from confounding is the major advantage of randomized trials over observational studies. Trials are still prone to other problems inherent in clinical research studies, such as misclassification, sampling variation, and limited external validity.

Table 8.6 Common reasons for null findings in randomized trials

Population	Study population not responsive to the treatment
	Inadequate number of study participants (low power)
Intervention	Insufficient dose or amount of the treatment
	Off-target effects of the treatment negate potential benefits
	Treatment has no true impact on the disease process
Outcomes	Selected outcomes do not capture the effects of the treatment
	Inadequate number of outcomes (low power)
	Imprecise measurements of the outcomes (low power)
Follow-up	Insufficient duration of follow-up
	High rate of dropout or switching (under intention-to-treat analysis)

8.9.5 Negative Trials

There are numerous reasons as to why so many randomized trials of promising therapies fail to demonstrate benefit (Table 8.6). Many flaws that arise in the design, conduct, and analysis of randomized trials tend to diminish the observed effects of the treatments under study, reducing the ability of the trial to detect the health impact of these treatments.

References

1. Wolfe RA, Ashby VB, Milford EL, et al. Comparison of mortality in all patients on dialysis, patients on dialysis awaiting transplantation, and recipients of a first cadaveric transplant. N Engl J Med. 1999;341(23):1725–30.
2. Global Use of Strategies to Open Occluded Coronary Arteries in Acute Coronary Syndromes Angioplasty Substudy I. A clinical trial comparing primary coronary angioplasty with tissue plasminogen activator for acute myocardial infarction. N Engl J Med. 1997;336(23):1621–8.
3. Pfeffer MA, Burdmann EA, Chen CY, et al. A trial of darbepoetin alfa in type 2 diabetes and chronic kidney disease. N Engl J Med. 2009;361(21):2019–32.
4. Ridker PM, Danielson E, Fonseca FA, et al. Rosuvastatin to prevent vascular events in men and women with elevated C-reactive protein. N Engl J Med. 2008;359(21):2195–207.
5. O'Brien PE, Dixon JB, Laurie C, et al. Treatment of mild to moderate obesity with laparoscopic adjustable gastric banding or an intensive medical program: a randomized trial. Ann Intern Med. 2006;144(9):625–33.
6. Fried LF, Emanuele N, Zhang JH, et al. Combined angiotensin inhibition for the treatment of diabetic nephropathy. N Engl J Med. 2013;369(20):1892–903.
7. Group ISS, Lundgren JD, Babiker AG, et al. Initiation of antiretroviral therapy in early asymptomatic HIV infection. N Engl J Med. 2015;373(9):795–807.
8. Weiss NS. All-cause mortality as an outcome in epidemiologic studies: proceed with caution. Eur J Epidemiol. 2014;29(3):147–9.
9. Cardiac Arrhythmia Suppression Trial I. Preliminary report: effect of encainide and flecainide on mortality in a randomized trial of arrhythmia suppression after myocardial infarction. N Engl J Med. 1989;321(6):406–12.

10. Weiss NS, Koepsell TD, Psaty BM. Generalizability of the results of randomized trials. Arch Intern Med. 2008;168(2):133–5.
11. Pitt B, Zannad F, Remme WJ, et al. The effect of spironolactone on morbidity and mortality in patients with severe heart failure. Randomized Aldactone evaluation study investigators. N Engl J Med. 1999;341(10):709–17.
12. Juurlink DN, Mamdani MM, Lee DS, et al. Rates of hyperkalemia after publication of the randomized Aldactone evaluation study. N Engl J Med. 2004;351(6):543–51.

Chapter 9
Misclassification

Summary of Learning Points

9.1 Misclassification results from errors in measuring the study data.

9.2 Non-differential misclassification describes errors that occur randomly or to a similar degree across a study population.

    9.2.1 Non-differential misclassification of the exposure occurs when errors in exposure measurements are similar among people with and without the outcome.

    9.2.2 Non-differential misclassification of the outcome occurs when errors in outcome measurements are similar among exposed and unexposed people.

    9.2.3 Non-differential misclassification of the exposure typically leads to attenuation of the observed relative risk.

9.3 Differential misclassification describes systematic errors in study measurements.

    9.3.1 Differential misclassification of the exposure occurs when errors in exposure measurements differ appreciably among people with and without the outcome.

    9.3.2 Differential misclassification of the outcome occurs when errors in outcome measurements differ appreciably across levels of the exposure.

    9.3.3 Differential misclassification may exaggerate the size of an association, dilute an association, or create false associations.

© Springer Nature Switzerland AG 2019

B. Kestenbaum, *Epidemiology and Biostatistics*,

https://doi.org/10.1007/978-3-319-96644-1_9

9.1 Definition of Miscalculation

It is often difficult for clinical research studies to obtain ideal measurements of the study data. Idealized, or "gold-standard" procedures for acquiring human study data are typically prohibitively expensive or impractical to perform in large populations. For example, a gold-standard procedure for measuring blood pressure is the insertion of a specialized catheter into a conduit artery to record pressure waveforms. However, this procedure is invasive, expensive, and not feasible to administer to a large number of people. In other instances, definitive measurements of study data may be impossible to obtain by *any* method. For example, there is no gold-standard procedure to measure the frequency and intensity of childhood bullying in a study that evaluates whether this exposure is associated with sleep disturbances. Consequently, most human research studies measure data using practical methods. Some examples are described in Table 9.1.

Misclassification refers to the false characterization of a study characteristic due to measurement error. Consider the example of hypertension (high blood pressure), for which the gold-standard method of measurement is invasive recording of pressure waveforms and the practical method is the use of a blood pressure cuff. In many instances, the results of these procedures will agree, because the cuff is a reasonably accurate tool for measuring blood pressure. Yet, in some instances, the blood pressure cuff will falsely classify a person's actual hypertension status, shown in Table 9.2.

The last two rows of the table demonstrate misclassification of hypertension by the blood pressure cuff, because the results of this practical test disagree with the actual hypertension status determined by the gold-standard method. Misclassification is also called *information bias*.

Any type of study data is subject to misclassification, including the exposure, outcome, and other study characteristics. Typically, misclassification of the expo-

Table 9.1 Practical and gold-standard methods for measuring human study data

Characteristic	Gold-standard measurement	Practical measurement
Heart failure	Adjudication of medical records	Hospital discharge codes
Aspirin use	Serum aspirin levels	Participant interview
Vitamin D levels	Mass spectroscopy	Immunoassay
Magnesium intake	Food diary with software analysis	One-day dietary recall
Muscle function	Cycle ergometer	Timed chair stands
Urinary protein excretion	24-h urine collection	Spot urine collection

Table 9.2 Correct and incorrect classification of hypertension status

Blood pressure cuff result (practical method)	Invasive waveform result (gold-standard method)	Classification of hypertension
Hypertension	Hypertension	Correctly classified
No hypertension	No hypertension	Correctly classified
Hypertension	No hypertension	Misclassified
No hypertension	Hypertension	Misclassified

sure or the outcome of a study has the greatest potential to undermine the ability of a study to obtain valid results. Since most studies do not include gold-standard measurements, there is often no way to "go back" and find out which measurements may have been misclassified. However, information regarding the accuracy of the procedures used to measure the study data can help infer whether misclassification is likely to have occurred. Such information can be combined with knowledge of the design and conduct of the study to deduce the expected impact of the misclassification on the study results.

9.2   Non-differential Miscalculation

9.2.1   Non-differential Misclassification of the Exposure

Example 9.1 Some studies have reported a link between marijuana use and depression, whereas other studies have found no such association. A hypothetical cohort study identifies 1000 college students who are initially free of major depression. Researchers determine the regular use versus nonuse of marijuana at the start of the study and then follow the students prospectively to assess the incidence of major depressive disorder.

First, consider an idealized situation in which the exposure and outcome are measured using gold-standard procedures. For example, a gold-standard method to determine marijuana use would be to measure cannabinoid levels in the urine on multiple occasions. Analogously, a gold-standard procedure to ascertain the study outcome, incident major depressive disorder, would be to conduct in-person examinations with trained therapists throughout the study. Table 9.3 presents hypothetical results obtained using gold-standard measurements of the exposure and outcome.

Given no misclassification of the exposure or outcome in this hypothetical study, regular marijuana use is associated with a two times higher incidence of major depression compared with no regular marijuana use.

As previously described, gold-standard measurements of human data are difficult to obtain. Study participants would likely be reluctant to undergo urinary drug testing, and such procedures might alter their behaviors. Similarly, conducting frequent follow-up examinations with medical professionals to assess depression would be prohibitively expensive in such a large study. Consider the impact of performing a more practical procedure to ascertain the exposure. The researchers

Table 9.3 Association of marijuana use with depression in the absence of misclassification

Regular marijuana use	Major depressive disorder		
	Yes	No	Total
Yes	50	450	500
No	25	475	500
	Relative risk = (50/500)/(25/500) = 2.0		

could administer questionnaires at the start of the study that inquire about recreational drug use, including marijuana. This method may introduce some degree of error in determining the participants' actual marijuana use. Suppose that 20% of regular marijuana users fail to report this behavior on the study questionnaires. Table 9.4 demonstrates the impact of this degree of exposure misclassification on the observed association with major depression.

To reflect the misclassified data, 20% of actual marijuana users are moved into the "no marijuana" group. In other words, the "no marijuana" group, defined by the questionnaire, now includes some actual marijuana users. The researchers conducting the study will observe and report the misclassified data on the right-hand side of the table and may be unaware that misclassification has occurred. Figure 9.1 illustrates the consequences of this exposure misclassification on the incidence and relative risk of major depressive disorder.

False reporting of "no marijuana use" among some true marijuana users will create a "nonuser" group that is intermixed with some actual marijuana users. The incidence of major depressive disorder in this mixed group will fall between that of true users and nonusers, yielding an attenuated relative risk of major depression

Table 9.4 Impact of misclassification of marijuana use on the observed relative risk

Results obtained using ideal measurements				Results observed using misclassified data			
	Depression				Depression		
	Yes	No	Total		Yes	No	Total
Marijuana	50	450	500	"Marijuana"	40	360	400
	10	90	100				
No marijuana	25	475	500	"No marijuana"	35	565	600
Relative risk = (50/500)/(25/500) = 2.0				Relative risk = (40/400)/(35/600) = 1.7			

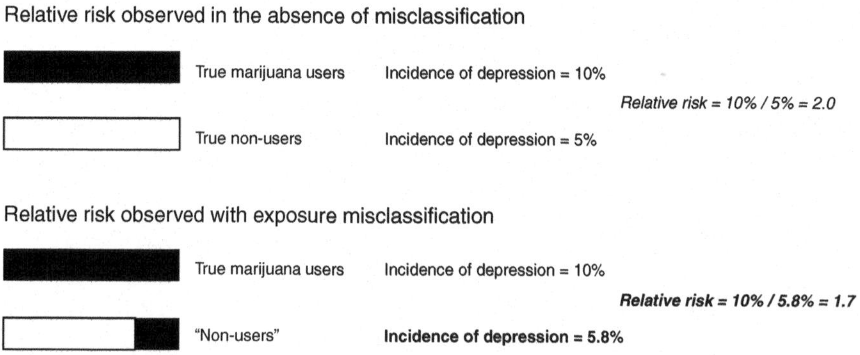

Relative risk observed in the absence of misclassification

True marijuana users   Incidence of depression = 10%

Relative risk = 10% / 5% = 2.0

True non-users   Incidence of depression = 5%

Relative risk observed with exposure misclassification

True marijuana users   Incidence of depression = 10%

Relative risk = 10% / 5.8% = 1.7

"Non-users"   **Incidence of depression = 5.8%**

Fig. 9.1 Relative risk observed under misclassification of the exposure

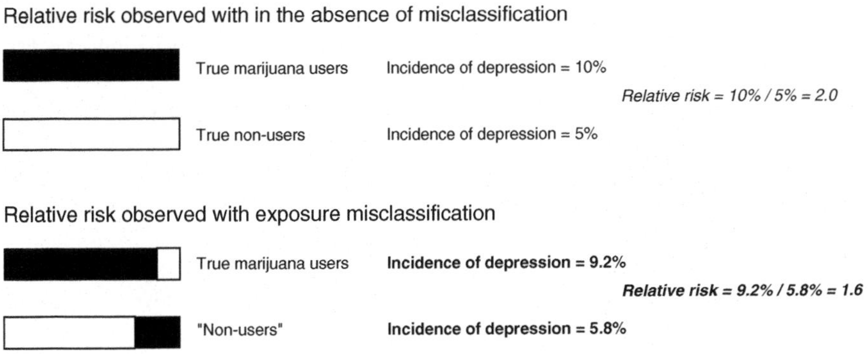

Relative risk observed with in the absence of misclassification

True marijuana users   Incidence of depression = 10%

Relative risk = 10% / 5% = 2.0

True non-users   Incidence of depression = 5%

Relative risk observed with exposure misclassification

True marijuana users   **Incidence of depression = 9.2%**

Relative risk = 9.2% / 5.8% = 1.6

"Non-users"   **Incidence of depression = 5.8%**

Fig. 9.2 Relative risk observed under bi-directional misclassification of the exposure

Absence of misclassification   Presence of misclassification

True marijuana users   "Marijuana users"

True non-users   "Non-users"

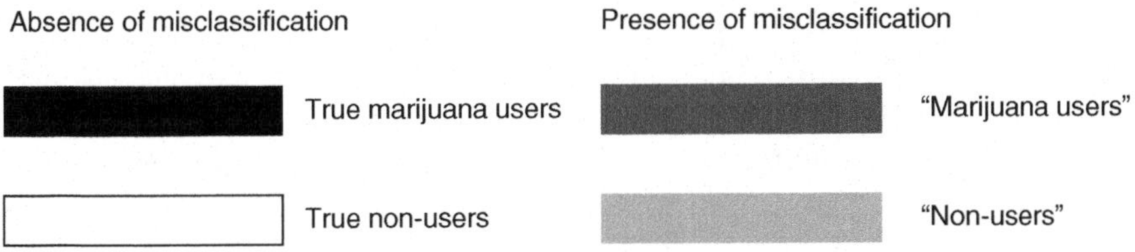

Fig. 9.3 Misclassification of the exposure diminishes contrasts in the study outcome

compared with the "ideal" relative risk theoretically obtained under ideal study measurements.

The above example considered only the possibility that some regular marijuana users falsely report this behavior on the questionnaire. It is also possible that some non-marijuana users may incorrectly report marijuana use in the study. Suppose that 10% of participants who are not actual marijuana users falsely report regular marijuana use on the study questionnaire. The impact of such bi-directional misclassification of the exposure is depicted in Fig. 9.2.

Misclassification of both marijuana users *and* nonusers will result in a further attenuation of the observed relative risk. The pattern of misclassification is causing the "marijuana use" and "nonuse" groups to blend together, muting the contrast in major depressive disorder between these two groups, shown in Fig. 9.3.

The above example assumed a similar degree of measurement error across the study population. Specifically, errors in classifying marijuana use were assumed to have occurred in equal proportions among participants who subsequently developed major depressive disorder during follow-up and those who did not. Such an assumption seems reasonable in this example, because there is no compelling reason to suspect that errors in reporting marijuana use at the start of the study would systematically differ according to the future development of depression.

Non-differential or *nonselective* misclassification of the exposure occurs when errors in exposure measurements are similar among people who incur and do not incur the outcome. Non-differential misclassification of the exposure typically leads to observing a relative risk that is closer to 1.0 than the "ideal" relative risk obtained using gold-standard measurements. This predictable attenuation of the relative risk is called *bias toward the null*.

Non-differential misclassification of the exposure commonly occurs with objective study measurements, such as quantitative laboratory assays, automated blood pressure readings, or genetic tests, provided that such procedures are applied consistently across the study population. Exposure measurements that require some degree of interpretation, such as imaging studies, microbiology colony counts, or biopsies, are also subject to non-differential misclassification if the person who is interpreting these tests is unaware of other participant data. Moreover, subjective procedures to measure exposures, such as questionnaires, can also lead to non-differential misclassification if there is little concern for systematic misreporting among the participants. Cohort studies often fit this description, because participants are typically unaware of their future disease status at the start of the study, when they report their exposures.

Example 9.2 Nuts are rich in antioxidants and other beneficial nutrients that may reduce the risk of certain chronic diseases. A cohort study examined the association of nut consumption with mortality among 118,962 men and women. The researchers quantified nut consumption by administering food frequency questionnaires every 2–4 years during the study. In adjusted analyses, the consumption of seven or more nut servings per week was associated with an estimated 20% lower risk of death compared with no nut consumption (relative risk 0.8).

The exposure in this study, nut consumption, may have been misclassified, because the food frequency questionnaire does not perfectly quantify actual nut consumption. There is no obvious reason to suspect that errors in the reporting of nut intake would systematically differ between people who subsequently died compared with those who survived. Consequently, misclassification of the exposure in this study was likely to have been non-differential, suggesting that the observed relative risk of 0.8 *underestimates* the "true" relative risk that would have been observed if nut consumption had been were measured perfectly. Importantly, misclassification is just one potential type of bias that may be impacting the results of this study. The observed association between nut consumption and survival could also be confounded by differences in the characteristics of people who tend to consume greater versus lesser servings of nuts.

9.2.2 Non-differential Misclassification of the Outcome

Returning to the hypothetical study of marijuana use and depression, what is the expected impact of misclassifying the study outcome, major depressive disorder? One practical method for ascertaining this condition is the Beck Depression Inventory (BDI), which is a standardized, self-administered psychometric test of depression and related symptoms. The researchers could administer this instrument annually to study participants to ascertain the incence of major depressive disorder over follow-up.

Table 9.5 Impact of overdiagnosing the study outcome

Results obtained using ideal measurements				Results observed using misclassified data			
	Depression				Depression		
	Yes	No	Total		"Yes"	"No"	Total
Marijuana	50	450	500	Marijuana	95	405	500
	45 ⟵						
No marijuana	25	475	500	No marijuana	73	427	500
	48 ⟵						
Relative risk = (50/500)/(25/500) = 2.0				Relative risk = (95/500)/(73/500) = 1.3			

The BDI does not perfectly classify major depressive disorder. For example, certain illnesses can increase the presence and severity of depression symptoms, yielding a BDI score that meets criteria for major depression when this condition is not truly present. Consider the possibility that 10% of participants who do not have a true diagnosis of major depressive disorder are falsely characterized as having this condition by the BDI. Table 9.5 demonstrates the impact of "overdiagnosing" major depressive disorder on the association of interest.

To reflect the misclassified data, 10% of participants without true depression are moved into the "depression" category. Stated another way, the "depression" group observed and analyzed by the researchers now includes some people without actual depression. The impact of this pattern of misclassification is, once again, to observe an attenuated relative risk of the outcome in comparison to the relative risk that would be obtained under ideal measurements.

This example assumed that errors in classifying major depressive disorder occurred to a similar degree among the marijuana users and nonusers in the study. It is possible that marijuana users tend to report more depression symptoms on the BDI compared with nonusers. However, such symptoms are more likely to reflect a true impact of marijuana use on depression, rather than systematic error of the BDI instrument in classifying this disorder. In other words, there is no compelling reason to suspect that the BDI would be more likely to create a *false* diagnosis of major depressive disorder specifically among marijuana users. Therefore, the assumption of non-differential misclassification of the outcome seems reasonable in this case.

The impact of non-differential misclassification of the outcome differs for the situation of underdiagnosis. For example, the BDI may also miss some true occurrences of major depressive disorder, particularly if the condition presents in an atypical manner. Table 9.6 depicts the consequence of missing 10% of actual instances of major depressive disorder in the study.

Somewhat surprisingly, underdiagnosis of the outcome has *no impact* on the observed relative risk when such errors occur in equal proportion among exposed and unexposed people.

Table 9.6 Impact of underdiagnosing the study outcome

Results obtained using ideal measurements			Results observed using misclassified data			
Depression				Depression		
Yes	No	Total		Yes	No	Total
Marijuana 50	450	500	"Marijuana"	45	455	500
→5						
No marijuana 25	475	500	"No marijuana"	22	478	500
→3						
Relative risk = (50/500)/(25/500) = 2.0			Relative risk = (45/500)/(22/500) = 2.0			

9.2.3   Summary of Non-differential Misclassification

Non-differential misclassification arises from non-systematic errors in measuring the study data. Specifically, non-differential misclassification of the exposure occurs when the amount and direction of error in exposure measurements are similar among people with and without the study outcome. Analogously, non-differential misclassification of the outcome occurs when the amount and direction of error in outcome measurements are similar across the exposure groups.

In most instances, non-differential misclassification will lead to bias toward the null, meaning that a study will observe and report a relative risk that is closer to 1.0 than the "ideal" relative risk that would be obtained under gold-standard measurements. The exception is for non-differential misclassification of the outcome in the setting of underdiagnosis, which does not impact the relative risk. Non-differential misclassification may dilute the size of observed associations, or may obscure the detection of true associations, but non-differential misclassification will *not* create false associations nor exaggerate the size of associations.

9.3   Differential Misclassification

9.3.1   Differential Misclassification of the Exposure

Example 9.3 Alcohol use during pregnancy adversely impacts fetal growth and development. A hypothetical case-control study examines the association of prenatal alcohol use with the occurrence of major structural birth defects. Researchers review birth record data to identify 30 case newborns who were diagnosed with a major birth defect and 90 control newborns who did not have a birth defect. The researchers then interview all of the study mothers to ascertain the frequency of alcohol use during pregnancy. Paradoxically, the study finds that any prenatal alcohol use is associated with a 20% *lower* risk of a major birth defect.

Could misclassification have played a role in this surprising result? The study outcome, a major birth defect, is typically obvious to diagnose and should be captured by
review of birth records. There is little reason to suspect misclassifcation of this outcome to any appreciable degree. On the other hand, the exposure, prenatal alcohol use,
is subject to misclassification, because interviews with study mothers may have led to
error in ascertaining this characteristic accurately. Gold-standard measurements of
prenatal alcohol use could theoretically be obtained by frequently monitoring blood
alcohol levels throughout pregnancy. However, such procedures would be impractical
and could alter the alcohol consumption habits of the participants.

The next step is to consider whether exposure misclassification in this study was
likely to have been non-differential or differential. Some non-differential misclassification of prenatal alcohol use may have occurred if the study mothers made general errors in recollecting their use of alcohol during pregnancy or if there was a
general tendency among study mothers to underreport prenatal alcohol use. Non-
differential misclassification of the exposure may have diluted the observed association between prenatal alcohol use and major birth defects to some degree.

Of potentially greater concern is the possibility that mothers of newborns who had
a major birth defect were *particularly likely* to withhold information about prenatal
alcohol use. In this case-control study, participants were aware of whether their child
had a major birth defect at the time of the interviews. Such knowledge may have
influenced some mothers of affected children to suppress information regarding their
alcohol use possibly due to feelings of guilt. Table 9.7 demonstrates the consequence
of underreporting prenatal alcohol use among six of the case mothers in the study.

Preferential underreporting of prenatal alcohol use among only six of the case
mothers grossly distorts the observed association of this exposure with major birth
defects. If prenatal alcohol use had been measured perfectly, then this exposure
would be associated with a 2.5 times higher odds of a major birth defect compared
to no prenatal alcohol use. In the presence of systematic misclassification of the
exposure, prenatal alcohol use is associated with a *lower* odds of a major birth defect.

Differential or *selective* misclassification of the exposure occurs when errors in
exposure measurements differ to an appreciable degree between people who have and

Table 9.7 Differential misclassification of the exposure

Results obtained using ideal measurements			Results observed using misclassified data		
	Birth defect			Birth defect	
	Yes	No		Yes	No
Prenatal alcohol use	10	15	"Prenatal alcohol use"	4	15
	↓				
	6				
No prenatal alcohol use	20	75	"No prenatal alcohol use"	26	75
Odds ratio = (10*75)/(15*20) = 2.5			Odds ratio = (4*75)/(15*26) = 0.8		

do not have the study outcome. In the above example, errors in measuring prenatal alcohol use were particularly pronounced among study mothers of newborns who had a major birth defect. This pattern of misclassification resulted in observing an association in the opposite direction of that obtained under ideal study measurements.

The differential misclassification described in this example illustrates the concept of recall bias previously described for case-control studies (Chap. 7). Recall bias can be avoided if the exposure can be measured before study participants are aware of the study outcome. For example, researchers conducting the study of prenatal alcohol use could have conducted interviews during later stages of pregnancy, but before the status of the newborn was known. Non-differential misclassification of the exposure may still occur under this appoach; however, the impact of this misclassification is predictable and unlikely to create a false association.

9.3.2   Differential Misclassification of the Outcome

Systematic errors in measuring the outcome of a study may occur if the procedures used for diagnosis are influenced by levels of the exposure. Recall the cohort study of the fictitious antibiotic, "supramycin," previously described in Example 6.3. Researchers conducting this study identified 100 patients with pneumonia who were treated with supramycin and a comparison group of 400 patients with pneumonia who were treated with amoxicillin. The researchers followed these patients over 4 weeks to compare the development of new rashes.

The participants and researchers in this study may have been aware of which antibiotic was received; blinding is not typically part of observational studies. It is possible that researchers' knowledge of the antibiotic type consciously or subconsciously influenced their determination of a rash. For example, preconceived concerns regarding possible side effects of supramycin may have prompted some of the researchers to overdiagnose innocuous skin lesion as "rash." Moreover, supramycin users may have been more likely to draw attention to skin lesions for diagnosis if they had misgivings about receiving this new antibiotic. Table 9.8 presents the impact of falsely classifying five normal skin lesions as "rash" among only the supramycin users.

Preferential misclassification of rash among only the exposed group (supramycin users) leads to observing an inflated relative risk compared with the "ideal" relative risk obtained under perfect study measurements.

9.3.3   Summary of Differential Misclassification

Differential misclassification arises from systematic errors in study measurements. Specifically, differential misclassification of the exposure occurs when the amount and direction of error in exposure measurements differ systematically between

Table 9.8 Differential misclassification of the outcome

Results obtained using ideal measurements				Results observed using misclassified data			
	Rash				"Rash"		
	Yes	No	Total		Yes	No	Total
Supramycin	10	90	100	Supramycin	15	85	100
	5 ←						
Amoxicillin	20	380	400	Amoxicillin	20	380	400
Relative risk = (10/100)/(20/400) = 2.0				Relative risk = (15/100)/(20/400) = 3.0			

people who develop or do not develop the outcome. Analogously, differential mis-classification of the outcome occurs when the amount and direction of error in outcome measurements differ systematically across the exposure groups. The impact of differential misclassification on the study results depends on the specific pattern of measurement error that has occurred. Differential misclassification can exaggerate an observed association, dilute an association, or create false associations. Careful appraisal of the study measurements is needed to estimate the direction of bias that may have resulted from differential misclassification. For this reason, differential misclassification is considered to be a more concerning type of bias than non-differential misclassification.

Note that the examples used throughout this chapter describe the consequences of misclassification for studies of binary exposures and binary outcomes. The impact of misclassification on more complex types of study data are beyond the scope of this book.

9.4   Assessment of Misclassification in Research Articles

The methods used to measure the exposure, outcome, and other study data are typically described in the *methods* section of a research article, following description of the study population. Importantly, research articles tend to use terminology that may suggest idealized measurements when, in fact, practical procedures were used to ascertain the study data. For example, a study comparing laparoscopic hernia repair versus open repair may assess the type of surgical procedure via telephone interview. An article reporting on these data may freely use the term, "laparoscopic hernia repair" throughout, rather than the reality, "all persons claiming to have undergone laparoscopic hernia repair by telephone interview."

The evaluation of misclassification in research studies is *subjective,* because there is often no way to go back and obtain gold-standard measurements of the study data. A useful approach for assessing the presence and impact of misclassification is to ask the following questions:

1. Based on data collection methods reported in the study, which characteristics are likely to have been misclassified (exposure, outcome, other data)?
2. Is the suspected misclassification likely to have been non-differential or differential?
3. What is the expected impact of the misclassification on the study results?

Appraisal of misclassification is facilitated by knowledge of the accuracy of the study measurements. For example, a number of prospective cohort studies have reported on the associations of specific prescription medications with long-term health outcomes. One procedure for ascertaining medication use in these studies called is the inventory method, in which study personnel ask participants to bring all of their medications to a study examination and then transcribe the prescription bottle labels. A validation study evaluated the accuracy of this procedure by comparing medication use reported by the inventory method to serum levels of the same medications [1]. The study found generally good agreement between the inventory method and serum detection for some medications, such as digoxin, but somewhat poor agreement for other drugs, such as aspirin. Statistical methods are available to address measurement error in the analyses if valid estimates of the direction and magnitude of error are available.

In summary, measurement error is ubiquitous in clinical research studies. The informed selection of appropriate procedures to measure the study data and the careful implementation of these procedures are important components of the design and conduct of research studies.

Reference

1. Smith NL, Psaty BM, Heckbert SR, Tracy RP, Cornell ES. The reliability of medication inventory methods compared to serum levels of cardiovascular drugs in the elderly. J Clin Epidemiol. 1999;52(2):143–6.

Chapter 10
Confounding

Summary of Learning Points

10.1 The presence of confounding obscures the interpretation of observational study data.

10.2 A confounding characteristic is associated with the exposure, associated with the outcome, and does not reside on the causal pathway of association.

10.3 Residual confounding refers to confounding by characteristics that were not measured in a study or characteristics that were measured with a considerable degree of error.

10.4 Confounding by indication occurs when the conditions that comprise the indication for a treatment confound the observed association of that treatment with outcomes.

10.5 Methods used to adjust for confounding include randomization, restriction, stratification plus adjustment, matching, and regression.

10.6 A consequential change in the size of an association after adjustment indicates the presence of confounding to a meaningful degree.

10.1 Confounding Obscure Understanding of Causal Relationships

Associations seen in observational studies that relate exposures to the occurrence of disease may or may not be indicative of causal relationships. The primary reason for uncertainty regarding causation in observational studies is the possibility of confounding. Conceptually, confounding occurs when other causes "stand in the way" of understanding a specific cause of interest. Specifically, confounding is present when characteristics other than the exposure of interest distort or bias the observed association of the exposure with disease.

© Springer Nature Switzerland AG 2019
B. Kestenbaum, *Epidemiology and Biostatistics*,
https://doi.org/10.1007/978-3-319-96644-1_10

The most definitive way to prevent confounding is to *assign* large numbers of people to specific exposures or treatments versus control procedures using a random process. However, randomized trials are often impractical for studying many potential risk factors for human diseases. Observational studies are essential tools for discovering novel causes of illness, appraising screening programs, understanding prognosis and countless other applications in medicine and public health. This chapter describes methods to identify confounding factors in observational studies and procedures to minimize their impact on the results.

Example 10.1 Researchers from a national cancer registry report an association of infectious mononucleosis with a higher incidence of Hodgkin lymphoma. This association could reflect direct carcinogenic effects of Epstein-Barr virus (the organism that causes mononucleosis) on B lymphocytes. On the other hand, people who contract mononucleosis may be more susceptible to other viral infections or have underlying differences in their immune functions that also increase the risk of lymphoma. In this instance, other causes "stand in the way" of establishing whether mononucleosis itself is a cause of lymphoma.

Example 10.2 A hypothetical observational study evaluates whether greater levels of usual physical activity are associated with a lower risk of hypertension. Researchers recruit 3000 participants who are initially free of hypertension, provide them with accelerometers to record usual physical activity levels over 4 weeks, and conduct annual follow-up exams to assess the occurrence of hypertension. The researchers divide physical activity levels into categories of "low" versus "high" based on a cut point of 8000 steps per day. Results are shown in Table 10.1.

Higher levels of usual physical activity are associated with a $(1.0–0.56) = 44\%$ lower incidence of hypertension. One interpretation of these findings is that greater amounts of physical activity *caused* the lower incidence of hypertension. If such a causal hypothesis were true, then next steps might include public health initiatives to increase the amount of physical activity in the population and experimental studies to probe possible mechanisms by which physical activity may reduce blood pressure. However, the lower incidence of hypertension observed among people who engaged in relatively high levels of physical activity could also have been caused by other characteristics. For example, people in the high physical activity group may have been younger, less likely to smoke, and more likely to follow a healthy diet compared with people in the low physical activity group. Stated another way, other characteristics may be *confounding* the observed association between usual physical activity levels and hypertension.

Table 10.1 Hypothetical study of usual physical activity levels and hypertension

Usual physical activity level	Number of participants	Cumulative incidence of hypertension
Low (≤8000 steps per day)	1800	18%
High (>8000 steps per day)	1200	10%
	Relative risk = 10%/18% = 0.56	

The presence of confounding does *not* imply that the study results are inherently false. People who engaged in relatively high levels of physical activity in this study truly experienced a 44% lower incidence of hypertension compared with people who engaged in relatively low levels. The possibility of confounding undermines the inference that greater physical activity levels itself is the *cause* of the lower incidence of hypertension, thereby altering the interpretation and consequences of the findings. For this reason, it is important to identify potential confounding characteristics in observational studies and attempt to correct for their distorting influence.

10.2 Evaluation of a Potential Confounding Characteristic

Confounding occurs when another characteristic is linked with both the exposure and the outcome of a study. Consider the possibility that the observed association between relatively high physical activity levels and a lower incidence of hypertension is confounded by sex. Such a possibility would require the potential confounder to be linked with both physical activity levels and hypertension within the study data, depicted in Fig. 10.1.

10.2.1 Confounding Characteristic Associated with the Exposure

The possibility of linkage, or association, between a potential confounding characteristic and the exposure is investigated by cross-tabulating the study data. Table 10.2 demonstrates cross-tabulation of the suspected confounder, sex, with the exposure, physical activity levels.

Fig. 10.1 Sex as a possible confounder in the study of physical activity levels

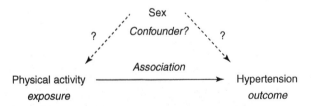

Table 10.2 Tabulation of a potential confounding characteristic with the exposure

	Exposure: usual physical activity level	
	Low (≤8000 steps per day)	High (>8000 steps per day)
Suspected confounder: sex	($N = 1800$)	($N = 1200$)
Female	540 (43%)	720 (57%)
Male	1260 (72%)	480 (28%)

Among the 1260 women in the study, 720 (57%) were in the high physical activity group. In contrast, only 28% of the men in the study were in the high physical activity group. Such a differential distribution of sex across the physical activity groups indicates a linkage, or association, between sex and the exposure within the study data.

It may be tempting to use statistical inference measures, such as *p*-values and confidence intervals, to evaluate associations of potential confounding characteristics with the exposure or outcome. However, inference measures are *not* useful for assessing the presence or magnitude of confounding and can be misleading in this application. *P*-values and confidence intervals relate findings obtained in a sample of people (the study population) to those from a theoretically infinite population of similar individuals. Yet, confounding arises from imbalances in the characteristics of the study participants themselves. To illustrate the limitation of statistical testing for evaluating the presence of confounding, consider a study of only ten people that also reports an association of relatively high physical activity levels with a lower incidence of hypertension. The researchers, concerned that this association may be confounded by sex, cross-tabulate their study data, shown in Table 10.3.

These results also demonstrate a sex discrepancy across physical activity levels within the study data. The nonsignificant *p*-value indicates uncertainty as to whether physical activity levels truly differ by sex in an infinitely large population of similar people. Such information is immaterial for assessing whether sex is confounding the results of this particular study.

Next, consider results of a very large study that also observes an association of relatively high physical activity levels with a lower incidence of hypertension. Table 10.4 cross-tabulates the suspected confounding characteristic, sex with physical activity levels.

The proportions of men and women are not quite identical across the physical activity groups in this study. However, such minor differences are unlikely to be appreciably distorting the observed association between physical activity levels and

Table 10.3 Association of sex with physical activity levels in study of ten people

	Exposure: usual physical activity levels	
Suspected confounder: sex	Low (≤8000 steps per day) (N = 6)	High (>8000 steps per day) (N = 4)
Female	2 (40%)	3 (60%)
Male	4 (80%)	1 (20%)
	P-value = 0.60	

Table 10.4 Association of sex with physical activity levels in study of 100,000 people

	Exposure: usual physical activity levels	
Suspected confounder: sex	Low (≤8000 steps per day) (N = 50,000)	High (>8000 steps per day) (N = 50,000)
Female	25,500 (51%)	24,500 (49%)
Male	24,500 (49%)	25,500 (51%)
	P-value <0.001	

hypertension. The significant *p*-value, which reflects the large number of participants, indicates that physical activity levels *are* likely to differ by sex, at least to some degree, in the underlying population from which these participants were selected. This fact does not impact whether the results of *this* study are meaningfully confounded by sex.

10.2.2 Confounding Characteristic Associated with the Outcome

Returning to the original study data, the next step for evaluating whether sex is a confounding characteristic is to cross-tabulate sex with the study outcome, incident hypertension, shown in Table 10.5.

The incidence of hypertension differs meaningfully by sex in this study: 19% of men but only 9% of women developed hypertension over follow-up. Such a large discrepancy indicates a link between sex and the study outcome.

Taken together, the data in Tables 10.2 and 10.5 establish that sex is associated with both the exposure and the outcome of the physical activity study. Stated another way, women in the study were more likely to engage in higher levels of physical activity *and* were less likely to develop hypertension, depicted in Fig. 10.2.

10.2.3 Confounding Characteristic Not on the Causal Pathway of Association

A final consideration is needed before concluding that sex is confounding the results of the physical activity study: this characteristic must *not* reside on the causal pathway of association. The causal pathway represents a conceptual mechanism, or group of mechanisms, that plausibly explains *how* an exposure of interest

Table 10.5 Tabulation of a potential confounding characteristic with the outcome

	Outcome: hypertension	
Suspected confounder: sex	Yes (N = 444)	No (N = 2556)
Female	112 (9%)	1148 (91%)
Male	332 (19%)	1408 (81%)

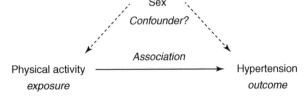

Fig. 10.2 Sex is associated with physical activity levels and hypertension

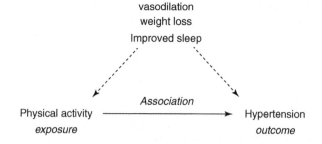

Fig. 10.3 Characteristics suspected to reside on the causal pathway of association

presumably impacts the study outcome. For example, possible mechanisms by which greater physical activity levels might reduce the risk of hypertension include arterial vasodilation, weight loss, and improved sleep, shown in Fig. 10.3.

The arrows in the causal diagram depict the presumed direction of the relationships under consideration. Greater amounts of physical activity are hypothesized to promote vasodilation, weight loss, and improved sleep, which subsequently reduce the incidence of hypertension. These characteristics would *not* be considered to represent confounders in this study; rather, they represent plausible *mediators* by which the exposure is suspected to influence the disease process. The causal pathway is informed from knowledge derived from other studies.

In contrast, consider the suspected directions of the relationships for sex, physical activity levels, and hypertension in Fig. 10.2. The presumed sequence is that a person's sex influences their likelihood of engaging in greater amounts of physical activity and also impacts their risk of developing hypertension. The alternative possibility that physical activity levels influence whether a person is biologically male or female is highly unlikely. For this reason, sex is *not* suspected to reside on the causal pathway of association in this study.

In summary, a confounding characteristic is defined as (1) associated with the exposure, (2) associated with the outcome, and (3) not suspected to reside on the causal pathway. The first two parts of this definition are evaluated by direct inspection of the study data. The third part is based on the conceptual relationships between the suspected confounder and the exposure and outcome of interest. Based on this definition, sex *is* likely to be confounding the association between physical activity levels and hypertension. The presence of confounding by sex creates uncertainty as to whether the observed association reflects the causal impact of physical activity itself on hypertension. Adjustment for sex, which forces the proportion of men and women to be equal in the two physical activity groups, would provide a clearer assessment of the association of interest.

Example 10.3 Hepatic steatosis is a disorder characterized by excess accumulation of fat within the liver. Researchers propose to test whether this condition is associated with the development of stroke. They plan to identify a cohort of people who have hepatic steatosis and a second cohort of people who do not have this condition.

Fig. 10.4 Causal diagram
for the study of hepatic
steatosis and stroke

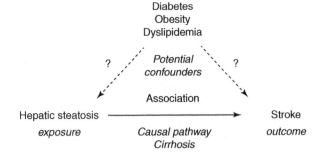

What characteristics might plausibly confound an observed association between hepatic steatosis and stroke?

People who have a diagnosis of hepatic steatosis may tend to also have other illnesses that could predispose to stroke. Knowledge of disease risk factors helps to inform a set of potential confounding characteristics. Based on information from other studies, known risk factors for stroke include hypertension, diabetes, obesity, smoking, and a sedentary lifestyle. Among these characteristics, diabetes, obesity, and a sedentary lifestyle are also risk factors for hepatic steatosis. These shared risk factors represent potential confounders of an association between hepatic steatosis and stroke, warranting inspection of the study data to assess potential linkages with the exposure and outcome.

Knowledge of disease mechanisms helps to delineate the presumed causal pathway of association. Hepatic steatosis can progress to cirrhosis (end-stage liver disease), which impairs the synthesis of certain blood clotting factors that can increase the risk of hemorrhagic stroke. Consequently, cirrhosis would be presumed to reside on the causal pathway between hepatic steatosis and stroke and would *not* be considered to represent a confounding characteristic in this study. Figure 10.4 depicts suspected confounding characteristics and those likely to reside on the causal pathway of association.

10.2.4 Evaluation of Confounding Characteristics in Research Articles

A strategy for appraising potential confounding characteristics in a research study is to begin with inspection of the *table of baseline characteristics*, which is often the first table of a research article. For cohort studies and randomized trials, the baseline characteristics table typically presents the exposure or treatment in the columns of the table and a list of participant characteristics in the rows. Table 10.6 demonstrates an example baseline characteristics table for the hypothetical study of physical activity levels and hypertension.

Table 10.6 Baseline characteristics table from study of physical activity and hypertension

	Exposure: usual physical activity level	
	Low (≤8000 steps per day) (N = 1800)	Low (≤8000 steps per day) (N = 1800)
Age (years)	63.7 ± 17.7	57.1 ± 19.2
Current smoking	286 (16%)	96 (8%)
Body mass index (kg/m²)	31.9 ± 5.2	27.8 ± 6.5
Alcohol use (drinks per day)	0.7 ± 0.4	0.7 ± 0.5
Dietary sodium (mg/day)	2918 ± 446.1	2847 ± 516.0

All values in the table expressed as mean ± standard deviation or number (percent)

Table 10.7 Baseline characteristics table from study of pervasive developmental disorder

	Outcome: developmental disorder	
	Yes (N = 1300 cases)	No (N = 4500 controls)
Child age in years (median)	5.4	4.9
Female	17%	17%
Years in general practice database (median)	3.3	3.4
Clinic visits per year prior to diagnosis (median)	5.4	4.0

These baseline data demonstrate notable differences in age, current smoking, and body mass index across the physical activity groups, highlighting these characteristics as possible confounding factors. Further assessment of potential linkages between these characteristics and the study outcome, hypertension, is needed to confirm or refute their confounding influence in this study. On the other hand, the frequency of alcohol use and the amount of dietary sodium intake are similar across the physical activity groups, suggesting that these characteristics are *not* relevant confounders here. Note that the study outcome, hypertension, is usually excluded from the table of baseline characteristics in cohort studies and clinical trials.

For case-control studies, participant characteristics are typically presented in relation to the study outcome. For example, Table 10.7 demonstrates baseline characteristics from the study of MMR vaccination and pervasive developmental disorder previously described in Chap. 7.

Age, sex, and years in the practice database are relatively similar among the case and control children, suggesting that these characteristics are *not* meaningful confounders in this study. There is some imbalance in the number of annual clinic visits, warranting assessment of whether this characteristic is also associated with the exposure, MMR vaccination.

Unfortunately, many research studies provide data for only one of the linkages needed to appraise confounding. For example, the study of physical activity levels may neglect to report associations of age, body mass index, and smoking with hypertension, the outcome. Analogously, the study of developmental disorder may fail to include the association of annual clinic visits with MMR vaccination status, the study exposure. In such instances, it is not possible to directly demonstrate associations of a suspected confounding characteristic with both the exposure and outcome of a study. However, knowledge from previous studies can be used to cast suspicion on certain characteristics as likely confounders. For example, older age and greater body mass index are established risk factors for hypertension, based on information from previous studies. Demonstration that these characteristics are associated with physical activity levels within the study data suggests that they may be confounding the observed association to a meaningful degree.

10.3 Residual Confounding

Residual confounding describes the presence of confounding by characteristics that are not collected in a study or characteristics that are measured with error. For example, the study of physical activity levels did not collect data regarding socioeconomic status or chronic pain symptoms. Such characteristics could confound the results if they were to influence both physical activity levels and the incidence of hypertension. Residual confounding can also arise from characteristics that are measured inaccurately. The data in Table 10.6 suggest similar amounts of dietary sodium intake between the high and low physical activity groups, seemingly excluding this characteristic as a meaningful confounder. However, common methods to quantify sodium intake, such as food frequency questionnaires and timed urine collections, have limitations in accuracy and precision, leaving open the possibility for residual confounding by differences in *actual* dietary sodium intake across the physical activity groups. Residual confounding may occur in studies that obtain unreliable data regarding comorbid illnesses from insensitive or non-specific diagnostic codes. Such studies may perform extensive adjustment for comorbidity; however, residual confounding by the actual presence and severity of these diseases remains a legitimate concern. The potential problem of residual confounding can be addressed by implementing more comprehensive procedures to accurately measure the study data, but *not by increasing the number of participants*. Residual confounding is the primary reason for uncertainty regarding causality in observational studies, because such studies cannot account for the presence and extent of *all* characteristics that may be confounding an observed association. Randomized trials, though not immune to their own inherent limitations, are usually the most definitive design for preventing confounding.

10.4 Confounding by Indication

Confounding by indication refers to a specific type of confounding seen in observational studies that examine the consequences of treatments or procedures. The concept is that the reasons for administering a treatment may themselves be related to the occurrence of the outcomes being studied.

Fig. 10.5 Confounding by indication in observational studies of loop diuretic use

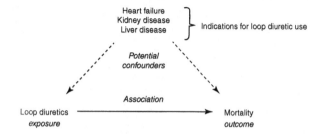

Example 10.4 Loop diuretics are medications that are used to reduce swelling due to heart failure, kidney dysfunction, or liver disease. Observational studies have reported that patients who receive loop diuretics experience greater risks of death and prolonged hospitalization compared with patients who do not receive these medications. If such associations represented the causal impact of loop diuretics on adverse outcomes, then use of these medications should be curtailed. On the other hand, associations between loop diuretic use and adverse outcomes may have been confounded. What characteristics are most likely to have confounded these associations?

Prescription medications have specific *indications* for use. In the United States, indications are regulated by the Food and Drug Administration and explicitly listed on the medication label. Loop diuretics are indicated to reduce swelling due to heart failure, kidney dysfunction, or liver disease, which are serious conditions that themselves may increase the risks of death and hospitalization. In other words, the specific indications for administering a loop diuretic are prime candidates for confounding, based on presumed linkages with the exposure and outcome, shown in Fig. 10.5.

10.5 Methods to Control for Confounding

Once suspected confounding characteristics have been identified, how should their distorting influence on the study results be controlled? For the study of usual physical activity levels and hypertension, the most definitive way to prevent confounding would be to randomly assign people to either low versus high levels of physical activity. Randomization would balance the proportions of men and women, as well as other characteristics across the physical activity groups. However, it would be challenging to conduct a trial that compels people to exercise and enforces this behavior over a long period of time. In non-randomized studies, methods to control for confounding include restriction, stratification plus adjustment, matching, and regression.

10.5.1 Method of Restriction

A simple procedure for removing the confounding influence of sex in the study of physical activity would be to exclude all of one sex from the study population. For example, removing all men from the study would leave no possibility for imbalances in sex across the physical activity groups and eliminate the possibility for confounding by this characteristic.

Restriction can be a useful method for convincingly removing the confounding influence of one or a small number of characteristics. However, restriction can substantially reduce the number of participants available for analysis, diminishing the power of a study to detect associations and reducing the external validity of the results. Removing all men from the physical activity study would greatly reduce study power and generate findings that apply exclusively to women. Many observational studies use restriction to prevent confounding by one or a small number of major disease risk factors. For example, a cohort study to investigate whether exposure to a specific manufacturing dye is associated with the incidence of bladder cancer may exclude smokers to eliminate the possibility of confounding by this strong risk factor for cancer.

In some instances, it may be necessary to use restriction to control for confounding when the possibility of residual confounding is unavoidable. For example, a community-based case-control study examined the association between exercise patterns and the risk of sudden cardiac death [1]. Of immediate concern is the possibility of confounding by the presence and severity of underlying heart disease, which could impair a person's ability to exercise and increase their risk of cardiac death. Measuring and adjusting for *all* aspects of cardiac disease, including the extent of coronary atherosclerosis, ventricular function, and underlying arrhythmias, would be exceedingly difficult. In this instance, the study excluded people who reported *any* known history of heart disease. The use of restriction in this example greatly reduced the potential for confounding by heart disease; however, some degree of residual confounding by clinically inconspicuous (subclinical) cardiac disease remains possible.

Restriction can also be used to control for confounding by indication in observational studies of medications or procedures. In Example 10.4, the use of a loop diuretic was found to be associated with mortality and prolonged hospitalization, yet these associations were suspected to be confounded by the conditions comprising the indication for a loop diuretic. Restricting the study population to people who have an indication for these medications will substantially reduce the possibility of confounding. To accomplish this, the researchers would first identify a group of patients who *all* have swelling due to heart failure, kidney dysfunction, or liver disease, such that the entire study population has an indication for a loop diuretic. The researchers would then classify participants as exposed versus unexposed based on whether or not they received a loop diuretic and assess associations of this exposure with relevant outcomes. Restriction by indication attempts to isolate the causal effects of a treatment by creating a more homogenous study population. Some residual confounding may persist under this design. Patients who receive loop diuretics may have more severe swelling or more extensive comorbidities compared with those who do not receive these medications.

10.5.2 Method of Stratification plus Adjustment

Instead of simply excluding all of one sex from the physical activity study, these groups can be temporarily separated for the purposes of analysis and then rejoined. *Stratification* describes the process of dividing a study population into smaller subgroups (strata) according to a specific characteristic. Table 10.8 presents data from the physical activity study stratified by sex.

Because each stratum consists of only one sex, there is no possibility for confounding by sex within either stratum. The unconfounded relative risks within each stratum can then be rejoined to create a summary relative risk, which is also not confounded by sex.

A simplified approach for combining the relative risks for men and women would be to calculate their average. However, a simple average would ignore differences in the relative numbers of people and outcomes within each stratum. A somewhat better method would be to weigh each relative risk by the proportion of people in the stratum. From Table 10.8, women comprised $(1260/3000) = 42\%$ of the study population and men comprised $(1740/3000) = 58\%$.

A simple combined or *summary relative* risk can be calculated as:

$$\text{Relative risk}_{\text{summary}} = \left(\text{relative risk}_{\text{women}} \times \text{weight}_{\text{women}}\right) + \left(\text{relative risk}_{\text{men}} \times \text{weight}_{\text{men}}\right)$$
$$\text{Relative risk}_{\text{summary}} = \left(0.64 \times 0.42\right) + \left(0.67 \times 0.58\right) = 0.66$$

The summary relative risk of 0.66 represents the association of higher physical activity levels with hypertension *after adjustment for sex*. Weighing each relative

Table 10.8 Association of physical activity levels with hypertension stratified by sex

Stratum one: women only ($N = 1260$)		
Physical activity level	Number of participants	Cumulative incidence of hypertension
Low	540	11%
High	720	7%
		Relative risk = 7%/11% = 0.64
Stratum two: men only ($N = 1740$)		
Physical activity level	Number of participants	Cumulative incidence of hypertension
Low	1260	21%
High	480	14%
		Relative risk = 14%/21% = 0.67

risk by the proportion of people in each stratum oversimplifies the more complex weighting procedures typically used in research studies but illustrates the concept of weighing and combining risks across strata.

The method of stratification plus adjustment produces a single summary association but ignores whether the size of the individual associations differ across strata. Based on the data in Table 10.8, the association between higher physical activity levels and hypertension was similar among women (relative risk = 0.64) and men (relative risk = 0.67). However, any similarities or differences in the size of associations across strata will be masked by combining these associations into a single value. The concept that the size of an association may differ according to another characteristic is called *effect modification, which is conceptually different from confounding.* Effect modification is discussed in Chap. 11.

The major advantage of stratification plus adjustment, compared to restriction, is that this procedure preserves the full study population, thereby maintaining study power and external validity. The sex adjusted relative risk of 0.66 was calculated using data from all 3000 study participants and applies to both men and women.

Stratification is a useful method for handling *binary* characteristics, such as biological sex, which can assume only two possible values. Stratification is more difficult to perform for continuous characteristics, such as age. Stratification by age would require dividing the study population into several age groups, for example, <50 years, 50–70 years, and >70 years, and then weighing and combining the relative risks across these groups. This process would leave open the possibility for residual confounding by small age differences within each stratum.

The primary disadvantage of stratification is the inability to control for many confounding characteristics simultaneously. For example, concurrent adjustment for age, sex, *and* smoking status using stratification plus adjustment would require the creation of numerous strata, each representing a unique combination of these characteristics:

Stratum	Age group (years)	Sex	Smoking status
1	<50	Men	Non-smokers
2	50–60	Men	Non-smokers
3	60–70	Men	Non-smokers
4	<50	Women	Non-smokers
5	50–60	Women	Non-smokers
6	60–70	Women	Non-smokers
7	<50	Men	Smokers
And so on			

Some of these individual strata may be very small and contain no hypertension outcomes, preventing their contribution to the calculation of a summary relative risk.

Stratification can also provide additional insight into the concept of confounding. Consider the mortality rates of two hypothetical countries. Country One represents a hypothetical nation with an impeccable healthcare system and an aging

Table 10.9 Comparison of mortality rates between two hypothetical countries

Country one		Country two		
People (millions)	Mortality rate (per 100,000)	People (millions)	Mortality rate (per 100,000)	Relative risk
10	17.9	10	8.6	2.08

Table 10.10 Comparison of mortality rates between two hypothetical countries by age

Country one			Country two			
Age group (years)	People (millions)	Mortality rate (per 100,000)	Age group (years)	People (millions)	Mortality rate (per 100,000)	Relative risk
0–30	0.5	2.0	0–30	7.0	3.9	0.52
30–50	1.0	4.0	30–50	1.5	7.3	0.55
50–70	1.5	9.3	50–70	1.0	22.0	0.42
>70	7.0	22.9	>70	0.5	51.0	0.44

population. Country Two represents a nation that lacks health infrastructure and has a low life expectancy. Overall mortality rates of the two countries are presented in Table 10.9.

Surprisingly, the mortality rate is considerably higher in the country with the reportedly superior healthcare system. Stratifying the mortality rates of the two countries by age helps to explain this apparently paradoxical finding, shown in Table 10.10.

The mortality rate in Country One is substantially lower than that of Country Two in every age category. These categories include all possible ages; no people were excluded.

The age distributions of the two countries are markedly different. Although advances in healthcare may have contributed to the relatively low mortality of older adults in Country One, this mortality still exceeds that of younger people in Country Two. The comparison of overall mortality rates allowed these age groups to mix together, thereby contrasting the mortality of relatively older people in Country One with relatively younger people in Country Two.

Stratifying the data by age with subsequent adjustment provides a fairer comparison of mortality rates, weighing and combining relative risks from each age category in Table 10.10:

	Country one	Country two	Total	
Age group (years)	People (millions)	People (millions)	People (millions)	Proportion of total
0–30	0.5	7.0	7.5	7.5/20.0 = 0.375
30–50	1.0	1.5	2.5	2.5/20.0 = 0.125
50–70	1.5	1.0	2.5	2.5/20.0 = 0.125
>70	7.0	0.5	7.5	7.5/20.0 = 0.375
Total	10.0	10.0	20.0	

$$\text{Relative risk}_{\text{summary}} = (0.52 \times 0.375) + (0.55 \times 0.125) + (0.42 \times 0.125) \\ + (0.44 \times 0.375) = 0.48$$

This age-adjusted relative risk is substantially different, and in the opposite direction, from the unadjusted relative risk of 2.08. Such a large change in the size of the association after age adjustment indicates the presence of strong confounding by age.

10.5.3 Method of Matching

Matching is another method used to control for confounding in observational studies. Unlike stratification, which is conducted after the study data have been collected, matching must be performed as part of the initial study procedures. The general goal of matching is to increase the degree of similarity in one or more suspected confounding characteristics across the exposure or outcome groups. Table 10.11 demonstrates the process of matching by sex and smoking status in the study of physical activity levels and hypertension.

Matching can be considered as an iterative process. Researchers would first identify an exposed person, defined by having relatively low physical activity levels and determine their sex and smoking status (person 1a). Next, they would find an unexposed person (high physical activity levels) who is of the same sex and has the same smoking status (person 1b). Repeating this procedure will create a study population in which the proportions of women and smokers will be balanced across the physical activity groups.

The above example illustrates the process of matching on the exposure in a cohort study. For case-control studies, which target groups of diseased and non-diseased individuals, matching is typically performed per the study outcome. Consider the case-control study of MMR vaccination and pervasive developmental disorder. The researchers first identified 1300 case children who were diagnosed with a developmental disorder. They next attempted to find up to five control children per case who were of similar age (within 1 year), shown in Table 10.12.

Table 10.11 Matching confounding characteristics by the exposure in a cohort study

Identify				Match			
Person	Exposure	Sex	Smoking	Person	Exposure	Sex	Smoking
1a	Low activity	Female	No	1b	High activity	Female	No
2a	Low activity	Male	Yes	2b	High activity	Male	Yes
3a	Low activity	Male	No	3b	High activity	Male	No
4a	Low activity	Female	No	4b	High activity	Female	No
And so on							

Table 10.12 Matching confounding characteristics to the outcome in a case-control study

Identify			Match		
Person	Outcome	Age	Person	Outcome	Age
1a	Developmental disorder	4.1 years	1b	No developmental disorder	4.2 years
2a	Developmental disorder	5.6 years	2b	No developmental disorder	5.4 years
3a	Developmental disorder	6.4 years	3b	No developmental disorder	6.3 years
4a	Developmental disorder	5.2 years	4b	No developmental disorder	5.5 years
And so on					

Matching suspected confounding variables according to the outcome can adequately address confounding; however, this procedure requires additional methods to control for the matching variables in the analyses. Conceptually, a confounding characteristic requires linkage with both the exposure and the outcome of a study. Breaking just one of these links is sufficient to control for the confounding influence of that characteristic.

There are no specific rules regarding the optimal number of matched individuals. Studies will typically select up to three to four matched persons per group depending on the number available for matching. Adding more controls beyond three to four per group has diminishing impact on statistical power, which describes the ability of a study to detect associations that are truly present.

Advantages of matching include the intuitive nature of the procedure and the potential to adjust for more than one confounding characteristics simultaneously. However, the use of matching to control for many characteristics will be limited by the number of available people who can be matched. Suppose researchers conducting the physical activity study decided to match on age, race, sex, smoking status, diabetes, and body mass index. This process would require finding unexposed individuals who are similar to exposed individuals with respect to *all* of these matching characteristics. Sufficient numbers of such people may not be available.

A specialized method to handle this situation is called propensity score matching. This procedure constructs a mathematical model to estimate the likelihood (probability) of the exposure based on a combination of characteristics. For example, a model could estimate the probability of engaging in relatively high levels of physical activity based on age, race, sex, smoking status, diabetes history, and body mass index. The researchers would then match each exposed person (low physical activity levels) to one or more unexposed people (high physical activity levels) according to a similar predicted probability of the exposure, thereby controlling for the set of potential confounding factors simultaneously. This procedure attempts to mimic that of a randomized trial for the measured study characteristics.

One limitation of matching is that this procedure must be included as part of the initial study design. Once a matched study population has been created, there is no way to "go back" and match on other characteristics. Another limitation is that the characteristics selected to be matching variables in case-control studies can no longer be evaluated as risk factors for the disease. For example, matching on sex in the study of pervasive developmental disorder will artificially create an equal proportion of boys with and without this disorder, precluding assessment of whether sex is a risk factor for the disease.

10.5.4   Method of Regression

Restriction, stratification, and matching have limited flexibility in adjusting for large numbers of confounding characteristics simultaneously. Regression is a mathematical procedure that fits complex models to the study data to control for confounding. Given satisfied assumptions of these models, regression can estimate the association of specific risk factors with disease after adjustment for many confounding factors. Regression is also capable of flexibly handling different types of study data, such as continuous and binary characteristics. For these reasons, regression is among the most popular methods used to control for confounding in research studies. Special care is needed in constructing these models, understanding their assumptions, and interpreting the output. Regression is covered in Chaps. 16 and 17.

10.6   Interpreting Results After Adjustment for Confounding

The physical activity study initially found that relatively high levels of usual physical activity were associated with a 44% lower incidence of hypertension (relative risk = 0.56). The investigation of sex as possible confounder revealed linkages among sex, physical activity levels, and hypertension and excluded the possibility that sex was residing on the causal pathway of association. Based on these considerations, sex was suspected to be confounding the observed association between physical activity levels and hypertension.

The method of stratification plus adjustment was used to control for the confounding influence of sex (Table 10.8). After adjustment for sex, relatively high physical activity levels were associated with only a 34% lower incidence of hypertension (relative risk = 0.66). This *meaningful change in the size of the relative risk after adjustment* implies that sex was confounding the original unadjusted study data.

There is no consensus rule as to how much change in an association after adjustment constitutes a "meaningful" change. A reasonable starting point is a 10% change.

$$\text{Change in relative risk}\left(\text{RR}\right) = \frac{\left(\text{RR after adjustment} - \text{RR before adjustment}\right)}{\left(\text{RR before adjustment}\right)} \times 100\%$$

Table 10.13 Unadjusted and adjusted associations of physical activity with hypertension

	Relative risk of hypertension[a]
Unadjusted	0.56
Adjusted for sex	0.66
Adjusted for sex, age, and smoking	0.79
Adjusted for sex, age, smoking, and alcohol use	0.80

[a]Relative risk compares >8000 versus ≤8000 steps per day of usual physical activity

For the example of sex:

$$\text{Change in relative risk} \left(RR \right) = \frac{\left(0.66 - 0.56 \right)}{\left(0.56 \right)} \times 100\% = 18\%$$

An 18% change in the size of the relative risk suggests that sex was confounding the unadjusted association of physical activity levels with hypertension to a meaningful degree.

Appraising differences in the size of associations in response to adjustment is readily applicable to the interpretation of results reported in research articles. Table 10.13 presents the association of higher physical activity levels with hypertension before and after adjustment.

Adjustment for sex results in a meaningful (18%) change in the unadjusted relative risk, suggesting that sex was confounding the unadjusted study data. Additional adjustment for age and smoking results in a further change in the relative risk from 0.66 to 0.79, corresponding to a 20% change. These adjusted data imply that age, smoking, or both characteristics in combination were meaningfully confounding the sex-adjusted relative risk. Further adjustment for alcohol use has little impact on the sex, age, and smoking-adjusted relative risk, suggesting negligible additional confounding by alcohol use on this association.

The association of physical activity levels with hypertension after adjustment for sex, age, and smoking suggests a somewhat lesser causal impact of this exposure on the incidence of hypertension than first suggested by the unadjusted study data. Removing the confounding influences of these characteristics yields a clearer picture of the effect of physical activity levels itself on hypertension. However, residual confounding remains an important concern, prohibiting conclusion that greater amounts of usual physical activity *cause* the lower risk of hypertension. Inference of a causal relationship requires consideration of other criteria, such as biological plausibility, which must be obtained from additional studies.

Reference

1. Lemaitre RN, Siscovick DS, Raghunathan TE, Weinmann S, Arbogast P, Lin DY. Leisure-time physical activity and the risk of primary cardiac arrest. Arch Intern Med. 1999;159(7):686–90.

Chapter 11
Effect Modification

Summary of Learning Points

11.1 Effect modification is defined as a differential impact of a treatment or exposure on the disease process.

11.2 Differences in the size of associations observed in studies may or may not represent a true differential impact of a treatment or exposure.

    11.2.1 Observed differences in the size of an association are more likely to represent an actual differential effect of an exposure or treatment on the disease if:

        11.2.1.1 The amount of difference in the association across subgroups is large.

        11.2.1.2 The subgroups contain sufficient numbers of people and outcomes.

        11.2.1.3 There is plausibility for the differential size of the association.

        11.2.1.4 The differential size of the association is replicated in other studies.

    11.2.2 Statistical measures estimate whether the differential size of an association likely exceeds chance but require careful interpretation in the context of multiple testing.

11.3 Effect modification addresses a fundamentally different concept than confounding.

11.4 The presence of effect modification on the additive scale suggests target populations that would receive the greatest benefits or harms from treatment.

Most research studies present measures of effect as an average obtained from the full study population. For example, a clinical trial compared two different treatment regimens for prostate cancer among 1917 men with newly diagnosed cancer [1].

© Springer Nature Switzerland AG 2019
B. Kestenbaum, *Epidemiology and Biostatistics*,
https://doi.org/10.1007/978-3-319-96644-1_11

Participants were randomly assigned to receive either androgen deprivation therapy (ADT) alone or combination therapy of ADT plus an androgen synthesis inhibitor and prednisolone. After 3 years, cancer-free survival was found to be 75% in the combination therapy group compared with 45% in the ADT-treatment alone group. This observed 30% difference in disease-free survival represents the *average* effect of the combined treatment regimen among all 1917 participants in the trial. It is possible that combination therapy has even greater benefits among certain groups of prostate cancer patients, such as men who have metastatic disease. On the other hand, combination therapy may be less effective in other groups, for example, men whose cancers are not hormone responsive. The relative safety of the two regimens may also differ across subgroups of patients.

Ideally, the differential impact of an exposure or treatment could be used to tailor the delivery of healthcare to people who would receive the greatest benefit while withholding treatments from others who may be most susceptible to harm. However, differences in the size of associations seen in research studies require cautious interpretation, because such differences may or may not represent a true differential impact of an exposure on the disease process.

11.1   Concept of Effect Modification

Effect modification occurs when the size of an association between exposure and outcome differs according to another characteristic. The size of the association may be quantified using any suitable measure of effect, such as relative risk, attributable risk, or the difference in mean values, described in Fig. 11.1.

Example 11.1 Recombinant tissue plasminogen activator (rtPA) is an intravenous medication used to dissolve blood clots and restore blood flow in the setting of acute stroke. In a pooled analysis of clinical trials, researchers compared the effectiveness of rtPA treatment among men and women with stroke [2]. The study found that rtPA therapy was associated with a 5% lower risk of stroke-related disability or death in men and a 25% lower risk of this outcome in women.

In this example, relative risk was used to quantify the size of the association between rtPA treatment and stroke outcomes. The size of this association was found to differ between men and women, suggesting effect modification by sex, depicted in Fig. 11.2.

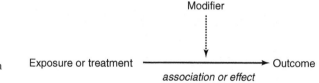

Fig. 11.1 Causal diagram of effect modification

Fig. 11.2 Sex modifies the impact of rtPA treatment on stroke outcomes

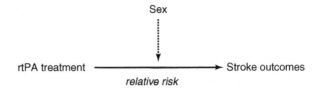

Table 11.1 Incidence of head and neck cancer by smoking and heavy alcohol use

Smoking	Heavy alcohol use	Incidence of head and neck cancer (cases per 100,000 person-years)
No	No	6.0
No	Yes	14.3
Yes	No	31.2
Yes	Yes	117.4

Several mechanisms may explain the differential impact of rtPA treatment on stroke outcomes by sex. Women tend to have higher circulating concentrations of plasminogen activator inhibitor-1, which is the target of rtPA therapy. Women also tend to present with less severe stroke symptoms than men, suggesting lesions that may be more responsive to rtPA treatment.

Example 11.2 Smoking and heavy alcohol use are risk factors for head and neck cancer, presumably acting through different mechanisms. Smoking is directly carcinogenic to squamous epithelial cells of the throat, and alcohol erodes the protective mucosal lining. Table 11.1 presents incidence rates of head and neck cancer by smoking and heavy alcohol use.

In the absence of heavy alcohol use, the additional incidence of head and neck cancer among smokers is 31.2 − 6.0 = 25.2 cases per 100,000 person-years. When combined with heavy alcohol use, smoking is associated with a much larger additional incidence of cancer: 117.4 − 14.3 = 103.1 cases per 100,000 person-years. These findings suggest that, on the additive scale, heavy alcohol use *modifies* the association between smoking and head and neck cancer.

A reciprocal interpretation of these data is that smoking modifies the association between heavy alcohol use and cancer. Such a mutual interaction between two (or more) risk factors is also called *synergy*. The incidence of head and neck cancer among people who have both risk factors is substantially greater than that predicted by their individual associations.

Example 11.3 Staphylococcus aureus is a colonizing bacterium that can cause life-threatening bloodstream infections. *Staphylococcus* bacteremia, defined by the presence of the organism in normally sterile blood, is among the most common invasive infections among hospitalized patients. A hypothetical clinical trial tests the effectiveness of a new vaccine to prevent *Staphylococcus* bacteremia. Eligibility criteria include age ≥50 years, hospitalization at a participating research center, and nasal colonization with *Staphylococcus aureus*. The researchers randomly assign

Table 11.2 Hypothetical trial of *Staphylococcus* vaccine among hospitalized patients

	Number of participants	New cases of staphylococcal bacteremia	Incidence of bacteremia (per 1000 hospital days)
Vaccine	5000	66	2.20
Placebo	5000	174	5.80
		Relative risk = 2.20/5.80 = 0.38	

Table 11.3 Hypothetical vaccine trial results stratified by steroid medication use

	Steroid medication use			No steroid medication use		
	Number of participants	New cases of bacteremia	Incidence rate[a]	Number of participants	New cases of bacteremia	Incidence rate[a]
Vaccine	800	18	3.75	4200	48	1.90
Placebo	800	20	4.17	4200	154	6.11
	Relative risk = 3.75/4.17 = 0.90			Relative risk = 1.90/6.11 = 0.31		

[a]Incidence rates expressed per 1000 hospital days

half of the study patients to receive the new vaccine and the other half to receive a placebo at the time of hospital admission. The outcome of the trial is the occurrence of staphylococcal bacteremia. Results are presented in Table 11.2.

Among all 10,000 trial participants, the new vaccine reduced the incidence of *Staphylococcus* bacteremia by (1.0–0.38) = 62% compared to placebo. The researchers conducting the study decide to next explore whether the new vaccine may be less effective at preventing bacteremia outcomes among patients who were concomitantly receiving oral steroid medications, because such medications can blunt vaccine responsiveness. Stratified trial data are presented in Table 11.3.

The new vaccine reduced bacteremia outcomes by only 10% among patients who were receiving steroid medications but by 69% among patients not taking these medications. These subgroup findings suggest that, on the relative risk scale, the new vaccine is less effective at preventing bacteremia outcomes among steroid medication users compared with nonusers.

11.2   Evaluation of Effect Modification

Contrasts in the size of an association observed in a research study may or may not represent a true differential impact of the exposure or treatment on the disease process. For one thing, the possibility of chance must be considered. Chance differences in the size of an association refer to the "natural" fluctuation that occurs when drawing a sample of people from a larger underlying population. Consider the 1600 trial participants who were receiving steroid medications as a random sample of *all* possible patients who receive steroid medications and would meet eligibility criteria for the trial, illustrated in Fig. 11.3.

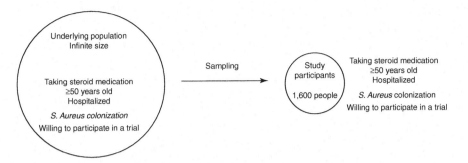

Fig. 11.3 Steroid medication users in the vaccine trial as a random sample

Diminished effectiveness of the *Staphylococcus* vaccine observed among this group of 1600 trial participants who were receiving steroid medications could represent a truly lesser impact of the vaccine among all similar people. On the other hand, contrast in the size of the vaccine effects seen in the trial could reflect a unique feature of these specific people.

11.2.1 Criteria for Assessing the Presence of Effect Modification

Differences in the size of an association seen in a research study are more likely to represent a true differential impact of an exposure or treatment on the disease if:

1. The amount of difference in the association across subgroups is large.
2. The subgroups contain sufficient numbers of people and outcomes for comparison.
3. The differential size of the association is plausible based on evidence from other studies.
4. The differential size of the association is replicated in other studies.

These criteria are identical to those previously described for appraising differences in treatment effects across subgroups in randomized trials (Chap. 8). Large differences in the size of an observed association are more likely to represent true differences, because chance and bias can produce only so much variation in well-conducted studies. For the hypothetical *Staphylococcus* vaccine trial, the differential size of the association between vaccination and bacteremia, comparing steroid medication users to nonusers was reasonably large: the vaccine reduced bacteremia outcomes by 69% among patients who were not receiving steroids but by only 10% among those who were receiving steroids.

The possibility for chance differences in the size of an association is reduced if the subgroups contain relatively large numbers of people and outcomes for comparison. Larger subgroups provide a more representative sample of the underlying population from which the participants were selected, reducing the amount of variation that can arise from sampling. The subgroup of steroid medication users in the vaccine trial was reasonably large (1600 people); however, the number of outcomes in this subgroup was modest (38 bacteremia cases).

Observed differences in the size of an association are more likely to reflect true differential effects of a treatment or exposure if the difference is supported by established biological, clinical, and/or scientific knowledge derived from other studies. The relatively weak effects of the new vaccine on preventing bacteremia among steroid medication users is supported by a body of existing evidence demonstrating blunted immune responsiveness due to steroid use.

In summary, the subgroup findings from the hypothetical trial suggest that the *Staphylococcus* vaccine *is* truly less effective for preventing bacteremia outcomes among patients who are receiving steroid medications. The observed difference in the relative risks is large; there are sufficient numbers of people in the subgroups; and there is biologic plausibility for a differential impact of the new vaccine on bacteremia outcomes. The best evidence to confirm a lesser impact of the new vaccine specifically among steroid medication users would come from additional studies that also observe this difference in treatment effect.

11.2.2 Statistical Considerations for Evaluating Effect Modification

Statistical inference measures, including *confidence intervals* and the *p-value for* interaction, can help appraise whether differences in the size of an association observed in a study exceed those expected from chance. To illustrate *how much* difference in the size of an association may be expected from chance alone, results of the hypothetical vaccine trial are presented in Table 11.4 stratified by the participant's astrological sign.

Table 11.4 Hypothetical vaccine trial results stratified by astrological sign

	Number of participants	Relative risk of *Staphylococcus* bacteremia comparing vaccine to placebo
All trial participants	10,000	0.38
Capricorn, "the goat"	833	0.43
Aquarius, "the water carrier"	833	0.37
Pisces, "the fish"	833	0.47
Aries, "the ram"	834	0.58
Taurus, "the bull"	833	0.31
Gemini, "the twins"	834	0.26
Cancer, "the crab"	833	0.49
Leo, "the lion"	833	0.26
Virgo, "the virgin"	834	0.29
Libra, "the scales"	833	0.27
Scorpio, "the scorpion"	833	0.30
Sagittarius, "the archer"	834	0.63

The new vaccine appears to be particularly effective at preventing bacteremia outcomes among participants whose astrological sign is Gemini (relative risk = 0.26) but considerably less effective among those whose sign is Sagittarius (relative risk = 0.63). These differences reflect the natural fluctuation *that arises from sampling variation alone*. An exposure or treatment is more likely to have a truly differential impact on the disease process if observed contrasts in the size of the association exceed that expected from chance.

11.2.2.1 Confidence Intervals

Confidence intervals (discussed in detail in Chap. 14) estimate an expected range of likely results in the theoretically infinite population from which the study participants were selected. Table 11.5 adds 95% confidence intervals to the subgroup analysis of the *Staphylococcus* vaccine trial.

Among the 1600 trial participants who were receiving steroid medications, the relative risk of bacteremia comparing the new vaccine to placebo is 0.90. The corresponding 95% confidence interval of (0.48–1.70) can be interpreted as: there is "95% confidence" that the relative risk of bacteremia, comparing the new vaccine to placebo, could be as low as 0.48 or as high as 1.70 in the theoretically infinite population of all steroid medication users who are similar to those in the trial. Among the 8400 trial participants who were not receiving steroid medications, the 95% confidence interval (0.23–0.43) can be interpreted as: there is "95% confidence" that the relative risk of bacteremia could be as low as 0.23 or as high as 0.43 in the theoretically infinite population of similar people who are not receiving steroid medications.

The 95% confidence interval for the relative risk in the no steroid medication use subgroup is considerably narrower than the corresponding interval in the steroid medication subgroup. The smaller number of participants who were receiving steroid medications provides less certainty as to the true relative risk in the underlying population of all similar people.

The 95% confidence intervals for the steroid medication use subgroups *do not overlap with one another*. The upper bound for the effect of the new vaccine among all similar steroid medication users is a (1.0–0.48) = 52% reduction in bacteremia outcomes. The lower bound for the effect of the vaccine among all similar people

Table 11.5 Hypothetical vaccine trial results stratified by steroid use with confidence intervals

	Steroid medication use			No steroid medication use		
	Number of participants	New cases of bacteremia	Incidence rate	Number of participants	New cases of bacteremia	Incidence rate
Vaccine	800	18	3.75	4200	48	1.90
Placebo	800	20	4.17	4200	154	6.11
	Relative risk = 3.75/4.17 = 0.90			Relative risk = 1.90/6.11 = 0.31		
	95% confidence interval (0.48–1.70)			95% confidence interval (0.23–0.43)		

who are not using steroid medications is a $(1.0–0.43) = 57\%$ reduction in bacteremia outcomes. These non-overlapping confidence intervals suggest that the observed contrast in the size of the relative risks exceeds that expected from chance.

11.2.2.2 *P*-value for Interaction

The *p*-value for interaction is a complementary statistical measure used to assess whether observed differences in the size of an association are likely to exceed chance differences. The *p*-value for interaction is defined as the probability of observing a specific difference in the size of an association, or an even larger difference, if no true difference in the size of the association exists in the underlying population. For example, the p-value for interaction comparing the relative risks across the steroid medication subgroups is 0.03. This *p*-value is interpreted as, "if the new vaccine were equally effective at preventing bacteremia outcomes among all similar steroid medication users and nonusers in the population, then the chance of observing these different relative risks, or an even larger difference in relative risks, is 3%." This relatively low p-value for interaction value suggests that the observed difference in relative risks across the steroid medication subgroups exceeds that expected from chance.

11.2.2.3 Multiple Testing

An important caveat for interpreting statistical inference tests is the number of tests performed on the same data. The above interpretations of the 95% confidence intervals and p-value for interaction assumed testing for differential effects of the *Staphylococcus* vaccine by only the use versus nonuse of steroid medications. Suppose the investigators decided to further explore whether the new vaccine might have differential effects on bacteremia outcomes by age, sex, white blood cell count, and the resistance patterns of the organism. In the context of multiple testing, the probability of observing one statistically significant contrast in the size of the vaccine effects for *any* of these comparisons is much greater than that for just a single comparison. As an analogy, there is a much greater chance of obtaining at least one six when rolling multiple dice compared to rolling just a single die.

Consider the p for interaction value of 0.03 for the difference in the size of the relative risks comparing steroid medication users to nonusers. In the context of testing for differences by only steroid medication use, this p-value is interpreted as a 3% probability of observing such a large difference, or an even larger difference, in relative risks due to chance. However, the same p for interaction value reflects a considerably greater than 3% chance of observing *any* such large difference in relative risks when additionally testing for contrasts by age, sex, white blood cell count, and *Staphylococcus* resistance patterns.

A common approach for handling multiple testing is to lower the p-value threshold for declaring statistical significance. As an extreme example, the threshold to declare significance in many genome-wide association studies, which perform up to ten million simultaneous inference tests, is 0.00000005. Ideally, higher levels of confidence should also be used for comparisons under multiple testing, such as 99% confidence intervals. In the absence of correction for multiple comparisons, statistical testing for effect modification may be unreliable.

Example 11.4 Glucosamine and chondroitin sulfate are dietary supplements used to treat osteoarthritis. A factorial design randomized trial assigned patients with knee osteoarthritis to receive either glucosamine, chondroitin sulfate, both treatments, or two placebos for 24 weeks [3]. The primary outcome of the trial was a 20% reduction in knee pain. Secondary outcomes included changes in perceived stiffness, function, and disability. At the end of the study, there were no significant differences in the primary outcome, or any of the secondary outcomes, among the treatment groups. The researchers next decided to explore whether the study treatments might have differential effects on the outcomes according to the severity of knee pain at the start of the trial. They found that combined treatment with glucosamine plus chondroitin sulfate was associated with a particularly great reduction in pain among participants who reported moderate to severe pain at baseline, shown in Table 11.6.

Do these results suggest a truly differential impact of glucosamine plus chondroitin sulfate treatment on pain specifically among people who have moderate to severe baseline pain? The observed difference in the size of the association is modest: combined treatment achieved a 79% reduction in pain among participants with moderate to severe baseline pain versus a 63% reduction among participants with mild baseline pain. These reductions are not substantially different from those observed in the respective placebo groups. There is no straightforward reason as to *why* the effects of these treatments would be particularly strong in the setting of greater pain; glucosamine and chondroitin sulfate are hypothesized to stimulate cartilage growth and reduce inflammation, which should provide pain relief across the spectrum of pain severity. The number of people with moderate to severe baseline pain who received both treatments was relatively small. Considering the criteria used to judge the presence of effect modification, the subgroup finding described in Table 11.6 is likely to be spurious. It would be premature to conclude that, among persons with moderate to severe baseline arthritis pain, there is particular benefit of glucosamine plus chondroitin sulfate treatment on that pain.

Table 11.6 Subgroup analysis from clinical trial of glucosamine plus chondroitin sulfate

	Placebo	Glucosamine	Chondroitin	Both treatments
Mild pain at baseline				
Number of participants	243	247	248	245
Proportion achieving 20% reduction in knee pain	62%	64%	67%	63%
Moderate to severe pain at baseline				
Number of participants	70	70	70	72
Proportion achieving 20% reduction in knee pain	54%	66%	61%	79%

The treatment effects reported in Table 11.6 were found to be statistically different across subgroups of mild versus moderate to severe baseline pain: p-value for
interaction =0.002. However, this statistical result was obtained in the context of
testing associations of four different treatment groups on a total of 14 different study
outcomes across subgroups of baseline pain. The effect of glucosamine plus chondroitin sulfate treatment did not differ according to the level of baseline pain for any
of the other study outcomes. In the context of multiple testing, and considering the
lack of other evidence to support a differential impact of combined treatment, this
statistical finding likely represents a false-positive result.

11.3   Effect Modification and Confounding Are Distinct Concepts

Effect modification and confounding are fundamentally different concepts that are
sometimes confused due to the seemingly analogous methods used for evaluation.
Confounding describes the distortion of an observed association by another characteristic, thereby obscuring whether the exposure of interest is likely to be a cause of
the outcome under study. Effect modification describes the differential impact of an
exposure or treatment on a disease process across levels of another characteristic.
The method of stratification is commonly used to investigate the presence of confounding and effect modification, but each concept requires a specific analysis and
a distinct interpretation of the stratified data.

Example 11.5 Researchers examine whether a newly discovered bone-derived protein is associated with osteoporosis. They measure the new protein in blood samples
collected from 170 older adults participating in a community-based cohort study.
All participants were initially free of osteoporosis at the start of the study and are
followed prospectively for the development of osteoporosis, assessed by annual
measurements of bone mineral density. Results are presented in Table 11.7.

The presence of the new bone-derived protein is associated with a 44% greater
relative incidence of osteoporosis. Could this association indicate a causal impact of
the new protein on the development of the disease? It is possible that the new protein promotes osteoporosis by enhancing bone turnover or impeding bone formation. On the other hand, characteristics of participants who had detectable levels of
the protein could themselves be predisposing to osteoporosis. For example, the new
protein may be more likely to be present among women, who have a substantially
higher risk of osteoporosis compared to men.

Table 11.7 Association of new bone-derived protein with osteoporosis

Bone-derived protein	New osteoporosis cases		Total	Cumulative incidence
	Yes	No		
Present	18	32	50	0.36
Absent	30	90	120	0.25
				Relative risk = 0.36/0.25 = 1.44

Table 11.8 Association of a new bone-derived protein with osteoporosis in women

| Bone-derived protein | New osteoporosis cases | | Total | Cumulative incidence |
	Yes	No		
Present	16	4	20	0.8
Absent	24	6	30	0.8
				Relative risk = 0.8/0.8 = 1.0

Table 11.9 Association of a new bone-derived protein with osteoporosis in men

| Bone-derived protein | New osteoporosis cases | | Total | Cumulative incidence |
	Yes	No		
Present	2	28	30	0.067
Absent	6	84	90	0.067
				Relative risk = 0.067/0.067 = 1.0

The method of stratification plus adjustment can be used to investigate the possibility of confounding by sex. Specifically, the study data can be stratified by sex to facilitate calculation of separate relative risks for women and men, shown in Tables 11.8 and 11.9.

The study population is divided into men and women only; no participants were excluded.

The relative risks in each stratum can be weighed and combined to obtain a sex-adjusted relative risk. Given that 50/170 = 29% of participants are women and 120/170 = 71% are men:

$$\text{Relative risk}_{summary} = \left(\text{relative risk}_{women}\ ^* \text{weight}_{women}\right) + \left(\text{relative risk}_{men}\ ^* \text{weight}_{men}\right)$$
$$\text{Relative risk}_{summary} = \left(1.0^*\ 0.29\right) + \left(1.0^*\ 0.71\right) = 1.0$$

The sex-adjusted relative risk of 1.0 differs substantially from the unadjusted relative risk of 1.44. Such a meaningful change after adjustment implies that sex was in fact (strongly) confounding the initial unadjusted association. After adjustment for sex, the presence of the new protein is no longer associated with the incidence of osteoporosis.

A second question is whether the new protein may have a differential impact on the incidence of osteoporosis by sex. The unadjusted relative risk of 1.44 represents the average association calculated among all 170 participants in the study, including women and men. Inspection of the stratified data reveals that the size of relative risk is equal among women (relative risk = 1.0) and men (relative risk = 1.0) implying no effect modification by sex.

In summary, stratification can be used to evaluate the presence and magnitude of confounding by comparing the adjusted association, obtained by stratification plus adjustment, with the unadjusted association. A meaningful change in the size of the association after adjustment suggests the presence of confounding. Stratification also is used to assess the presence of effect modification *by comparing the size of the stratum-specific associations with one another.* Large differences in the size of an association across strata suggest a true differential impact of an exposure or treatment on the study outcome. However, additional criteria for judging effect modification should also be considered, including the possibility for chance differences in the size of the observed association and plausibility for the differential size of the association.

In this example, sex was found to be a strong confounder, but not an effect modifier, of the association between the new bone-derived protein and osteoporosis. In any study, a characteristic may act as a confounder, an effect modifier, both, or neither.

11.4   Effect Modification on the Relative and Absolute Scales

Effect modification is broadly defined as a difference in the size of an association across different groups of people. The interpretation of effect modification, if it is truly present, depends on the scale of the measurement used to quantify size. Table 11.10 presents 5-year cumulative incidence rates of cardiovascular disease among people treated and not treated with a statin medication. The data are stratified by the presence versus absence of chronic kidney disease, a condition characterized by particularly high rates of cardiovascular disease.

First, consider the differential impact of statin treatment on the incidence of cardiovascular disease outcomes using relative risk as the measure of effect.

$$\text{Relative risk in general population} = \text{Incidence}_{\text{statin}} / \text{Incidence}_{\text{no statin}} = 3.0 / 5.0 = 0.6$$

$$\text{Relative risk in chronic kidney disease} = \text{Incidence}_{\text{statin}} / \text{Incidence}_{\text{no statin}}$$
$$= 16.0 / 20.0 = 0.8$$

Based on this difference in relative risks, statin treatment appears to be more effective for preventing cardiovascular disease in the general population (1.0–0.6 = 40% relative reduction) compared to the chronic kidney disease population (1.0–0.8 = 20% relative reduction).

Next, consider differential associations of statin treatment with the incidence of cardiovascular disease using attributable risk as the measure of effect.

Table 11.10 Incidence of cardiovascular disease by statin treatment

	Five-year cumulative incidence of cardiovascular disease (per 100)	
	General population	Chronic kidney disease
Statin treatment	3.0	16.0
No statin treatment	5.0	20.0

$$\text{Attributable risk general population} = \text{Incidence}_{\text{statin}} - \text{Incidence}_{\text{no statin}}$$
$$= 3.0 - 5.0 = -0.2 \text{ per } 100$$

$$\text{Attributable risk chronic kidney disease} = \text{Incidence}_{\text{statin}} - \text{Incidence}_{\text{no statin}}$$
$$= 16.0 - 20.0 - 0.4 \text{ per } 100$$

When attributable risk is used to quantify the size of the associations, statin treatment is associated with a greater reduction in cardiovascular disease incidence in the population with chronic kidney disease. Which interpretation is correct?

Both assessments are "correct" but demonstrate contrasting interpretations of effect modification depending on the scale used to quantify the association of interest. Differential associations of statin treatment with cardiovascular disease outcomes on the relative risk scale suggest diminished cardiovascular benefit for an individual with chronic kidney disease. Several mechanisms may explain a weaker impact of statin treatment on cardiovascular outcomes in chronic kidney disease patients, including the emergence of non-cholesterol-mediated pathways of disease, such as vascular calcification and endothelial dysfunction, which are not targeted by statin therapy.

Yet, the differential impact of statin therapy on cardiovascular disease measured on the additive (attributable risk) scale suggests that this treatment will prevent more cardiovascular outcomes when administered to the chronic kidney disease *population*, among whom cardiovascular disease rates are highest. This concept can be appreciated through the number needed to treat, which is the reciprocal of attributable risk:

$$\text{Number needed to treat or harm} = 1 / \text{absolute value} \left(\text{attributable risk}\right)$$

Treating $(1/0.04) = 25$ people who have chronic kidney disease with a statin would be expected to prevent one cardiovascular disease outcome. In contrast, $(1/0.02) = 50$ people from the general population would need to be treated with a statin to achieve a similar benefit. This example highlights the importance of assessing effect modification on the additive scale if the intention is to identify target populations that are likely to receive the greatest benefits (or harms) from a treatment or intervention.

References

1. James ND, de Bono JS, Spears MR, et al. Abiraterone for prostate cancer not previously treated with hormone therapy. N Engl J Med. 2017;377(4):338–51.
2. Kent DM, Price LL, Ringleb P, Hill MD, Selker HP. Sex-based differences in response to recombinant tissue plasminogen activator in acute ischemic stroke: a pooled analysis of randomized clinical trials. Stroke. 2005;36(1):62–5.
3. Clegg DO, Reda DJ, Harris CL, et al. Glucosamine, chondroitin sulfate, and the two in combination for painful knee osteoarthritis. N Engl J Med. 2006;354(8):795–808.

Chapter 12
Screening and Diagnosis

Summary of Learning Points

12.1 Screening refers to the early detection of disease, before signs or symptoms are present; diagnosis refers to the identification of disease during the clinical presentation.

12.3 Qualities of diseases appropriate for screening include:

    12.3.1 Early recognition of the disease should provide benefit.

    12.3.2 The disease is harmful if left untreated.

    12.3.3 The disease should have a preclinical phase that can be detected by screening.

12.4 Qualities of tests appropriate for screening or diagnosis include:

    12.4.1 Validity – the ability of a test to detect true disease, as determined by a gold standard.

        12.4.1.1 Sensitivity and specificity describe the probability of having a positive or negative test given gold-standard evidence of the disease status.

        12.4.1.2 Positive and negative predictive values describe the probability of having or not having a diseae given a specific test result.

        12.4.1.3 Predictive values depend on the frequency of the disease in the tested population.

    12.4.2 Reliability describes the ability of a test to produce the same result consistently.

12.5 ROC curves describe the tradeoff between sensitivity and specificity for continuous tests.

12.6 Some studies of screening are subject to specific biases:

    12.6.1 Referral bias is caused by differences in the characteristics of screened versus unscreened individuals.

    12.6.2 Lead time bias is caused by adding extra low-risk time to the screened group when comparing survival among people whose disease was or was not screen-detected.

© Springer Nature Switzerland AG 2019
B. Kestenbaum, *Epidemiology and Biostatistics*,
https://doi.org/10.1007/978-3-319-96644-1_12

12.6.3 Length bias sampling is caused by preferential screen detection of mild disease.

12.7 Primary, secondary, and tertiary preventions are treatments intended to prevent disease.

12.7.1 Primary preventions are designed to prevent the initial development of disease.

12.7.2 Secondary preventions are designed to treat early stages of disease detected by screening.

12.7.3 Tertiary preventions are designed to prevent complications of known diseases.

12.8 Risk factors, even those strongly associated with a disease, often function poorly as clinically useful predictors of disease incidence.

Alice is a 45-year-old woman who has a positive screening mammogram. She asks her physician about the chance of this being actual breast cancer. The mammogram is 90% sensitive and 90% specific for detecting breast cancer, and the prevalence of breast cancer in her age group is approximately 1%. What is the probability that Alice has breast cancer?

Screening and diagnostic tests are important clinical tools for identifying diseases at an early stage and promoting treatments that benefit tested individuals. Careful implementation and interpretation of these tests are needed to avoid clinical confusion, restrain healthcare costs, and prevent unnecessary complications caused by follow-up procedures that are prompted by positive test results.

12.1   General Principles of Screening and Diagnosis

Consider a "typical" disease process from biological onset through clinical outcome, depicted in Fig. 12.1.

Screening refers to the early detection of disease during the *preclinical phase*, in which a disease exhibits biological manifestations but has not yet caused recognizable symptoms or signs. For example, colonoscopy is a procedure used to identify

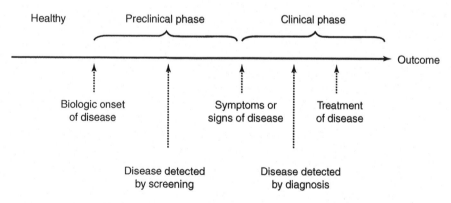

Fig. 12.1 Detection of disease by screening and diagnostic tests

adenomatous polyps or early-stage colorectal cancers, which only infrequently cause pain or perceptible symptoms. The use of colonoscopy to detect such lesions among asymptomatic people is an example of screening. Analogously, the use of mammography to detect early breast cancers among women such as Alice, who does *not* have apparent signs or symptoms of cancer, is also an example of screening.

Diagnosis refers to the identification of disease during the *clinical phase*, in which symptoms or signs of a disease are already present at the time of testing. For example, adenomatous polyps can enlarge over time and cause gastrointestinal bleeding. The use of colonoscopy to determine the cause of such bleeding is an example of a diagnostic test. Analogously, performing a skin biopsy to determine the cause of a suspicious appearing red nodule on a person's forehead is also an example of a diagnostic test, which is intended to confirm the diagnosis of skin cancer or suggest an alternative cause of the lesion.

12.2   Utility of Testing

Screening and diagnostic tests are often judged by their ability to predict disease. The capability of a test to reliably determine the presence or absence of disease (test validity) is undoubtedly important. Yet, validity alone is insufficient justification for administering a test. Additional information, often derived from many studies, is needed to appraise the *utility* of a screening or diagnostic test, including:

1. The prevalence of the disease in the tested population
2. The benefits of detecting and treating the disease at an earlier stage
3. The potential harms incurred from diagnostic procedures that follow a positive test

Example 12.1 A blood test that detects cancer-specific proteins and mutations in cell-free DNA was developed to identify latent solid tumors [1]. The test was administered to 1005 patients who had a confirmed diagnosis of a localized solid organ cancer and 812 cancer-free individuals. The test returned a positive result in 70% of the patients with cancer and less than 1% of the controls.

These findings demonstrate an impressive ability of the new test to accurately identify occult cancers. Additional steps are necessary to determine the potential health impact of the new test. For example, if the test were administered to a healthy population, about how many positive results would be expected? This number will depend on the prevalence of occult solid cancers among the tested population and the residual inaccuracy of the test. If the test is positive, what diagnostic procedures should be performed next? Presumably a positive test would prompt more comprehensive studies, such as imaging tests and biopsies. The costs and inherent risks of such procedures must be considered with the knowledge that some or many people who are referred for testing will not have actual disease (false positives). If the presence of early stage occult cancer is confirmed, can existing treatments alter the course of such nascent disease?

It would be difficult for a single study to address *all* of these questions. For example, consider a hypothetical randomized trial to determine the health impact of the new screening test. Such a trial could randomly assign large numbers of people to either receive the new test or follow currently accepted cancer screening guidelines and then compare outcomes, such as cancer-specific mortality, between these groups. However, a randomized study that evaluates clinical outcomes would be limited by requirements for a very large sample size and long duration of follow-up. On the other hand, the impact of the new screening test could be addressed by separate studies that determine the frequency of a positive test among different populations, evaluate potential adverse effects of the diagnostic procedures that follow a positive test, and assess the ability of existing cancer therapies to improve outcomes among people who have early disease detected by screening.

12.3 Qualities of Diseases Appropriate for Screening

12.3.1 Early Recognition of the Disease Should Provide Meaningful Benefit

The detection of a disease by a screening or diagnostic test should provide benefit for the tested individual, the healthcare system, or society. For example, the identification of adenomatous polyps by colonoscopy prompts removal of these precancerous lesions, thereby providing direct benefit to the patient. Analogously, the measurement of serum cholesterol levels can provide benefit to the tested individual by promoting treatment with lipid-lowering medications that reduce cardiovascular risk. The benefits of testing need not be limited to the successful treatment of a disease. Prenatal screening to identify chromosomal abnormalities, such as trisomy 21, does not yet lead to curative therapies but provides important information for parents. In other instances, the justification for testing may be less certain.

Example 12.2 Chronic kidney disease (CKD) affects approximately 11% of American adults and is associated with greater risks of cardiovascular disease and premature death. Several studies have identified genetic polymorphisms (inherited variations in DNA sequence) that are associated with the incidence of CKD. The most strongly associated genetic variants can be aggregated into a "gene score" that improves the ability to predict the incidence of the disease beyond traditional risk factors.

The association of the CKD gene score with the development of the disease, in and of itself, does not clarify whether the test should be administered to screen for this condition. CKD represents a heterogeneous group of disorders for which there is no specific treatment. It may be tempting to surmise that early identification of CKD could promote more rigorous medical care, such as frequent blood pressure monitoring and dietary counseling, which might delay the onset of the disease. However, the impact of such procedures on the development and consequences of CKD is uncertain. The benefits of performing the gene test are ambiguous; such information could promote unnecessary follow-up procedures, increase patient anxiety, and/or encourage the use of unproven or harmful treatments.

12.3.2   Screening Tests Should Target Diseases that Have Potentially Serious Consequences

Screening tests typically focus on diseases that are harmful if left untreated. For example, phenylketonuria is a rare genetic disorder caused by the inability to metabolize the amino acid phenylalanine. Failure to recognize this condition before the development of recognizable symptoms can lead to severe cognitive disabilities among affected children. The early detection of phenylketonuria by a specialized blood test prompts elimination of phenylalanine from the diet, which can prevent the serious consequences of the disease.

12.3.3   Diseases Targeted by Screening Require a Preclinical Phase

Screening tests detect biological manifestations of disease that are present before clinical signs or symptoms are apparent. In this regard, colorectal cancer represents an ideal disease for screening because progression from biological onset to clinical presentation typically occurs over many years and because the testing procedure, colonoscopy, can detect both polyps, a preclinical phase of colorectal cancer, and early colorectal cancer itself. On the other hand, it would be difficult to screen for acute infectious diseases, such as influenza, because clinical signs of the disease occur rapidly after biological onset.

12.4   Qualities of Tests Appropriate for Screening or Diagnosis

To achieve widespread use, a test should be easy to administer, inexpensive, and safe. Many blood tests and imaging studies satisfy these criteria, such as the prenatal triple screen test for detecting fetal genetic abnormalities and the chest X-ray to screen for tuberculosis. These tests are easy to administer, relatively inexpensive, and cause little harm. Beyond these general qualities, screening and diagnostic tests are evaluated based on their validity and reliability.

12.4.1 Validity

Validity, or accuracy, refers to the ability of a test to identify actual disease, as determined by a *gold-standard method*. Gold-standard procedures to confirm the presence or absence of a disease are typically invasive, expensive, and/or impractical to apply to large populations. For example, the validity of mammography for detecting breast cancer is typically judged by comparison with breast biopsy plus histologic examination, which is the gold-standard method for diagnosis. For some diseases, the gold-standard diagnostic procedure may be expert opinion. For example, heart failure is a clinical condition defined by a constellation of symptoms, signs, and characteristic responses to treatment. The validity of a diagnostic test for heart failure, such as blood levels of B-type natriuretic peptide (BNP), is assessed by comparison with the expert opinion of physician adjudicators who carefully review the available medical data.

12.4.1.1 Sensitivity and Specificity

Sensitivity and specificity are measures of test validity. Sensitivity is defined as the proportion of people who test positive among all people who have gold-standard evidence of disease.

$$\text{Sensitivity} = \frac{\text{number of people with gold-standard evidence of disease who test positive}}{\text{number of people with gold standard evidence of disease}}$$

For example, the sensitivity of mammography for detecting breast cancer is 90%. This value is interpreted as "90% of women who have biopsy-proven breast cancer will have a positive mammogram."

Specificity is defined as the proportion of people who test negative among all people with gold-standard evidence for the *absence* of disease.

$$\text{Specificity} = \frac{\text{number of people with gold-standard absence of disease who test negative}}{\text{number of people with gold-standard absence of disease}}$$

The specificity of mammography for detecting breast cancer is also about 90%. This value is interpreted as "90% of women who have biopsy-proven absence of breast cancer will have a negative mammogram."

Sensitivity and specificity values are determined from studies that include gold-standard measurements of disease status. The sensitivity and specificity of mammography were obtained from studies that evaluate this procedure among separate groups of women who have biopsy-proven breast cancer and biopsy-proven absence of breast cancer.

Sensitivity and specificity can be considered to represent fixed characteristics of a test that remain consistent across populations or vary to only a small degree. The 90% sensitivity and 90% specificity of mammography for detecting breast cancer may differ to some extent among older women, or women who have dense breast tissue; however, these values will be regarded as constant for the purposes of calculating predictive values (see Sect. 12.4.1.2, below).

The 90% sensitivity of mammography represents the chance of obtaining a positive mammogram among women who have biopsy-proven breast cancer. Yet, the results of breast biopsy are typically unknown at the time of testing. To interpret the results of screening and diagnostic tests in a clinical context, the probability of having disease given a positive or negative test result is needed.

12.4.1.2 Positive and Negative Predictive Values

Predictive values describe the probability of having actual disease given the results of a test. Unlike sensitivity and specificity, which are presumed to represent fixed values of a specific test, *positive and negative predictive values vary greatly according to the frequency of the disease in the tested population*. Predictive values are calculated from the sensitivity and specificity of a test *combined with the pretest probability of the disease*.

The pretest probability of disease is *estimated* from the context of testing. For screening tests, which are administered to people without recognizable symptoms or signs of a disease, the pretest probability is estimated by the *prevalence of the disease* among similar people in the population. Consider the use of ultrasonography to screen for testicular cancer among men ages 25–35-years-old. The pretest probability of the disease would be the prevalence of testicular cancer among all similarly aged men in the population.

For diagnostic tests, which are administered to people who already have suggestive signs or symptoms of a disease, the pretest probability is estimated by the unique aspects of the clinical presentation, including the nature of the symptoms, findings on physical examination, the results of related tests, and the judgment of the caregiver. In the context of diagnostic testing, the pretest probability of disease is typically much greater than that of screening. Consider the use of ultrasonography as a diagnostic test for testicular cancer among men who present with a solitary scrotal mass. The pretest probability of disease in this setting is estimated from unique aspects of the clinical presentation, including the size and quality of the mass and the presence versus absence of palpable lymph nodes. The ultrasound test may have the same sensitivity and specificity for detecting testicular cancer but markedly different positive and negative predictive values for identifying the disease depending on the context of testing.

The calculation of positive predictive values (PPV) and negative predictive values (NPV) can be demonstrated using a 2 × 2 table, in which gold-standard evidence of a disease is entered into the columns of the table and the test results are entered in the rows, shown in Table 12.1.

Table 12.1 Predictive values of a screening or diagnostic test

	Gold-standard evidence of disease		Total
	Yes	No	
Test positive	a	b	a + b
Test negative	c	d	c + d

Table 12.2 Predictive value of mammography as a screening test

	Gold-standard evidence of breast cancer		Total
	Yes	No	
Positive mammogram			
Negative mammogram			
Total	10	990	1000

$$\text{PPV} = \frac{\text{number of people with gold-standard evidence of disease who test positive}(a)}{\text{number of people who test positive}(a + b)}$$

Positive predictive value is the probability of having actual disease given a positive test.

$$\text{NPV} = \frac{\text{number of people with gold-standard absence of disease who test negative}(d)}{\text{number of people who test negative}(c + d)}$$

Negative predictive value is the probability of not having actual disease given a negative test.

To demonstrate the calculation and interpretation of predictive values, consider the original problem regarding the probability that Alice, a 45-year-old woman with a positive screening mammogram, has actual breast cancer. The sensitivity and specificity of mammography for detecting breast cancer are each 90%, and the prevalence of breast cancer in her age group is about 1%.

The first step for calculating predictive values is to estimate the pretest probability of disease. In this instance, mammography is used as a screening test, because Alice has no signs or symptoms of breast cancer at the time of testing. The pretest probability of disease in the context of screening is estimated by the prevalence of breast cancer among similar women in the population. Based on data from other sources, the prevalence of breast cancer among symptom-free women without a history of breast cancer in Alice's age group is given to be 1%. This pretest probability could be further refined, based on information about Alice's other cancer risk factors, such as a family history or genetic markers, if such data were available.

The pretest probability of disease is entered into the 2 × 2 table by first creating a total population of any size – 1000 is a reasonable round number – and then filling in the column totals, shown in Table 12.2.

Table 12.3 Predictive value of mammography as a screening test

| | Gold-standard evidence of breast cancer | | Total |
	Yes	No	
Positive mammogram	Sensitivity = 90% $(10 \times 0.9) = 9$		
Negative mammogram		Specificity = 90% $(990 \times 0.9) = 891$	
Total	10	990	1000

Table 12.4 Predictive value of mammography as a screening test

| | Gold-standard evidence of breast cancer | | Total |
	Yes	No	
Positive mammogram	9	99	108
Negative mammogram	1	891	892
Total	10	990	1000

Given an estimated 1% prevalence of actual breast cancer in Alice's age group, approximately 10 of 1000 asymptomatic women who undergo screening mammography will actually have cancer. The next step is to use the sensitivity and specificity characteristics of mammography to calculate the proportions of women who will test positive and test negative, shown in Table 12.3.

Based on the 90% sensitivity of mammography, 90% of women who have actual breast cancer will test positive. Analogously, based on the 90% specificity of mammography, 90% of women who do not have actual breast cancer will have test negative. The remaining cells in the table can then be completed from the above data, shown in Table 12.4.

Alice has a positive screening mammogram. The probability that she has actual breast cancer is the positive predictive value (PPV) of the test:

$$\text{PPV} = \frac{\text{number with gold-standard evidence of disease who test positive}\,(a)}{\text{number who test positive}\,(a+b)}$$
$$= 9/108 = 8.3\%$$

Given a positive screening mammogram, Alice has about an 8% chance of having actual breast cancer.

What if Alice has a negative mammogram? The probability that she has actual breast cancer given a negative test is the negative predictive value:

$$\text{NPV} = \frac{\text{number with gold-standard absence of disease who test negative}\,(d)}{\text{number who test negative}\,(c+d)}$$
$$= 891/892 = 99.9\%$$

Given a negative mammogram, Alice has a 99.9% probability of *not* having actual breast cancer.

The following steps summarize the procedure for calculating predictive values:

- Create a 2 × 2 table containing an arbitrary number of tested individuals, such as 1000.
- Estimate the pretest probability of the disease and enter into the column totals of the table.
- Apply the sensitivity and specificity of the test to calculate true positives and true negatives.
- Complete the remaining cells of the table.

Example 12.2 A company develops a new high-resolution imaging procedure for detecting breast cancer. The company reports the new test to be "extremely accurate," with 98% sensitivity and 95% specificity. A large health maintenance organization decides to deploy the new test to screen for breast cancer in 10,000 asymptomatic, 40–50-year-old female patients. Given an estimated 1% prevalence of breast cancer among asymptomatic women in this age group, how many false-positive tests would be expected?

The first step is to enter the estimated 1% pretest probability of breast cancer in a table representing the 10,000 women referred for testing, shown in Table 12.5.

Next, the sensitivity and specificity of the new test are applied to the data, shown in Table 12.6.

Among 10,000 asymptomatic women who undergo the new test, 495 without actual breast cancer would be expected to test positive (false positives). A positive screening test is likely to prompt a follow-up breast biopsy, which is invasive and expensive.

The above example highlights the difficulty in testing populations that have an inherently low prevalence of a disease: *the specificity of a test must be extremely high to prevent many false-positive results.* The 95% specificity of the new breast cancer test was inadequate for preventing a large number of false-positive results

Table 12.5 Predictive value of a new screening test for breast cancer

| | Gold-standard evidence of breast cancer | | |
	Yes	No	Total
Positive test			
Negative test			
Total	100	9900	10,000

Table 12.6 Predictive value of a new screening test for breast cancer

| | Gold-standard evidence of breast cancer | | |
	Yes	No	Total
Positive test	Sensitivity = 98% (100 × 0.98) = 98	**495 false positives**	593
Negative test	2	Specificity = 95% (9900 × 0.95) = 9405	9407
Total	100	9900	10,000

Table 12.7 Classification of test results

	Gold-standard evidence of disease	
	Yes	No
Positive test	True positives	False positives
Negative test	False negatives	True negatives

Table 12.8 Predictive value of mammography as a diagnostic test

	Gold-standard evidence of breast cancer		
	Yes	No	Total
Positive mammogram			
Negative mammogram			
Total	400	600	1000

Estimated frequency of disease based on clinical presentation = 40%

when the test was administered to a low-risk population (prevalence of disease = 1%). The problem of false-positive tests is particularly applicable to screening because the prevalence of disease among asymptomatic people is typically very low. Administering the new test to women with an inherently higher risk of breast cancer, such as women who have a first-degree relative with breast cancer, would reduce the number of false-positive tests at the expense of some increase in the number of false-negative tests.

Each cell in the 2 × 2 table of test results can be classified as true positives, true negatives, false positives, or false negatives, shown in Table 12.7.

Example 12.3 Ruth is a 45-year-old woman who has a positive screening mammogram. She asks her physician about the chance of this being actual breast cancer. Ruth was referred for mammography because of a suspicious breast mass that has doubled in size over the past 6 months. The mass is 1.5 cm in diameter, firm, and non-tender. Assume that mammography is about 90% sensitive and 90% specific for detecting breast cancer in women with a similar lesion.

In this example, mammography is used as a *diagnostic* test because Ruth has clinical findings suggestive of breast cancer at the time of testing. In the context of diagnostic testing, the pretest probability of disease is estimated from the clinical presentation of the tested individual, including the history of the illness, physical examination findings, and the judgment and experience of the caregiver. Given Ruth's presenting signs and symptoms, a reasonable estimate of her pretest probability of breast cancer is about 40%. The suspicious mass might be cancer but could also be caused by a benign condition, such as a cyst or fibrous tissue. To calculate the positive and negative predictive values of Ruth's diagnostic mammogram, the pretest probability of disease is first recorded in the columns of the 2 × 2 table, shown in Table 12.8.

Among 1000 hypothetical patients with a similar clinical presentation, about 40% are estimated to have actual breast cancer. Next, the 90% sensitivity and specificity of mammography, which are considered to represent fixed values of this test for detecting breast cancer, are applied to the data, shown in Table 12.9.

Table 12.9 Predictive value of mammography as a diagnostic test

| | Gold-standard evidence of breast cancer | | |
	Yes	No	Total
Positive mammogram	Sensitivity = 90% $(400 \times 0.9) = 360$	60	420
Negative mammogram	40	Specificity = 90% $(600 \times 0.9) = 540$	580
Total	400	600	1000

Estimated frequency of disease based on clinical presentation = 40%

$$PPV = \frac{\text{number with gold-standard evidence of disease who test positive} (a)}{\text{number who test positive} (a + b)}$$

$$= 360 / 420 = 86\%$$

Given Ruth's clinical presentation and a positive diagnostic mammogram, the probability that she has actual breast cancer is 86%.

How would a negative mammogram be interpreted in the context of Ruth's presentation?

$$NPV = \frac{\text{number with gold-standard absence of disease who test negative} (d)}{\text{number who test negative} (c + d)}$$

$$= 540 / 580 = 93.1\%$$

Given a negative mammogram, Ruth has a 93% probability of not having actual breast cancer. A negative mammogram in the setting of Ruth's high-risk clinical presentation still leaves some uncertainty as to the presence of actual cancer and warrants close follow-up and possibly additional testing.

12.4.1.3 Likelihood Ratios

A complementary approach to addressing screening and diagnostic testing problems is the use of *likelihood ratios*. Likelihood ratios combine sensitivity and specificity characteristics of a test in a manner that allows easy conversion of pretest probabilities into posttest probabilities.

$$\text{Likelihood ratio positive} = \text{sensitivity} / (1 - \text{specificity})$$

$$\text{Likelihood ratio negative} = (1 - \text{sensitivity}) / \text{specificity}$$

Note that likelihood ratios include only the sensitivity and specificity of a test, *not* the pretest probability of the disease, which must be estimated from the context of testing. Likelihood ratios are typically plotted using a nomogram to expedite calculation of posttest disease probabilities for any given test, shown in Fig. 12.2.

Fig. 12.2 Likelihood ratio nomogram

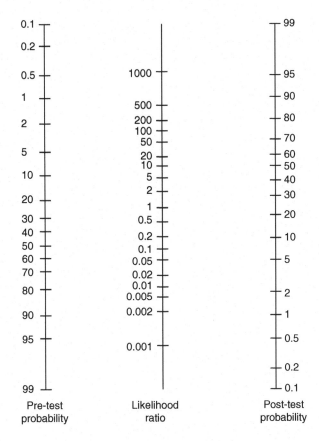

Analogous to the calculation of predictive values, the first step for using likelihood ratios is to estimate the pretest probability of disease. The pretest probability serves as the starting point on the left-hand column of the nomogram. If the test returns a positive result, use a straight line or ruler to connect the pretest probability of disease with the positive likelihood ratio in the middle column (positive likelihood ratios are the values >1.0). The resultant point in the posttest probability column represents the probability of disease given a positive test. If the test result is negative, connect the pretest probability of disease with the negative likelihood ratio for the test (negative likelihood ratios are the values <1.0). The resultant point on the posttest probability column represents the probability of disease given a negative test. A list of likelihood ratios for common tests is presented at the end of this chapter (Table 12.16).

Example 12.4 An 8-year-old boy presents to his pediatrician with a sore throat, runny nose, and fever of 3 days' duration. He has some tender anterior cervical lymph nodes and redness in the back of his throat, but no visible exudates. The boy's father is concerned about the possibility of strep throat and asks for a rapid strep test.

It is first useful to consider general aspects of the disease in question and qualities of the proposed diagnostic test. Streptococcal pharyngitis is a bacterial infection that can be serious if left untreated. Potential complications, albeit uncommon, include retropharyngeal abscess, rheumatic fever, and glomerulonephritis. A valid test confirming the presence of this condition would motivate antibiotic treatment, which is typically curative. A negative test would also be helpful for ruling out streptococcal pharyngitis as a cause of the illness, preventing unnecessary antibiotic treatment and suggesting other possible causes, such as a viral infection. The rapid strep test has reasonably good validity for detecting streptococcal pharyngitis: the sensitivity of the test is 90% and the specificity is 95%. These sensitivity and specificity values correspond with a positive likelihood ratio of 18 and a negative likelihood ratio of 0.1.

The pretest probability of disease in the context of diagnostic testing is estimated from aspects of the clinical presentation. Streptococcal infection is often accompanied by a sore throat, fever, and cervical lymphadenopathy, which are present in this case. On the other hand, strep pharyngitis is a relatively uncommon cause of upper respiratory infections. Moreover, strep infections are not typically associated with a runny nose and often includes exudative lesions, which are absent in this case. Based on these considerations, the estimated pretest probability of disease in this child is probably around 10%. As demonstrated here, the pretest probabilty of disease in the context of diagnostic testing is typically an estimate based on the clinical experience of the caregiver who is incorporating the clinical data.

Figure 12.3 demonstrates the use of the likelihood ratio nomogram to calculate the posttest probability of disease if the rapid strep test is positive. The line connects the estimated 10% pretest probability of disease with the positive likelihood ratio of 18 for the rapid strep test.

If the rapid strep test is positive in this child, then the probability of streptococcal pharyngitis is about 67%. Based on the potential seriousness of the condition and the availability of relatively safe and effective treatment, a positive rapid strep test would warrant antibiotic treatment.

Figure 12.4 demonstrates the use of the likelihood ratio nomogram to determine the posttest probability of disease if the rapid strep test is negative. The line connects the estimated 10% pretest probability of disease with the negative likelihood ratio of 0.1 for the test.

Given a negative test, there is a <1% probability of streptococcal pharyngitis. If this child has a negative rapid strep test it would be reasonable to withhold antibiotics, schedule a follow-up visit, and reassure the boy's father that streptococcal infection is unlikely. In summary, the administration of the rapid strep test is warranted in this situation because the results of the test are likely to influence subsequent care and provide benefit to the tested individual.

12.4.2 Reliability

Reliability refers to the ability of a test to produce the *same result consistently*. Reliability is also called *repeatability* or *precision*. The ability of any screening or diagnostic test to detect disease will be diluted if the test generates highly variable results. Table 12.10 presents results of the rapid strep test administered to the same three people over 7 days.

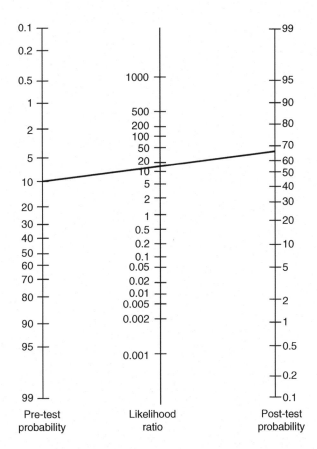

Fig. 12.3 Likelihood ratio nomogram for a positive streptococcal antigen test

The rapid strep test returns generally consistent results within the same individual, whether positive or negative; however, some variability is present. The observed within-person variation could be caused by differences in specimen collection and handling and/or inherent imprecision of the test itself. Similar considerations apply to the use of the potassium hydroxide test to diagnose cutaneous fungal infections. This test may yield different results when repeated on the same person due to differences in sample preparation and/or the subjective opinion of the tester who is looking under the microscope.

Note that reliability specifically describes the fluctuation inherent in a test and *not* the capability of the test to detect actual gold-standard disease (validity), depicted in Fig. 12.5.

12.4.2.1   Coefficient of Variation

The reliability of a test can be determined by repeating the test multiple times in succession. Several different measures are used to quantify and report the result of test reliability. For continuous tests, a common measure is the coefficient of variation.

$$\text{Coefficient of variation} = (\text{standard deviation of test / mean value of test}) \times 100\%$$

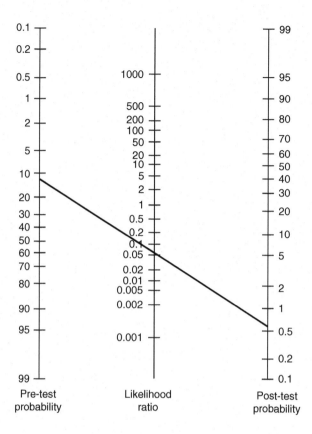

Fig. 12.4 Likelihood ratio nomogram for a negative streptococcal antigen test

Table 12.10 Reliability of the rapid streptococcal antigen test

	Person 1	Person 2	Person 3
Monday	Negative	Negative	Positive
Tuesday	Negative	Negative	Positive
Wednesday	Negative	Positive	Positive
Thursday	Negative	Negative	Positive
Friday	Negative	Negative	Positive
Saturday	Positive	Negative	Positive
Sunday	Negative	Negative	Negative

A lower coefficient of variation indicates a more reliable test; values <10% imply reasonably good reliability. Table 12.11 demonstrates calculation of the coefficient of variation for serum measurements of prostate-specific antigen (PSA) a test used to detect cancer, within the same person over a 24-h period.

The coefficient of variation of 9.1% includes biological fluctuation in circulating PSA levels over the course of a day and the inherent variation of the laboratory assay. The specific laboratory component of variation could be distinguished by performing the PSA test multiple times in succession on the same blood sample.

Fig. 12.5 Validity and reliability of screening and diagnostic tests

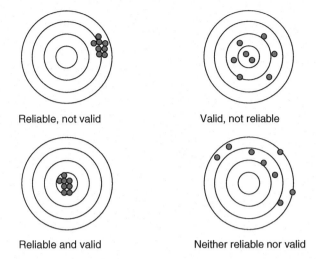

Reliable, not valid   Valid, not reliable

Reliable and valid   Neither reliable nor valid

Table 12.11 Reliability of the prostate-specific antigen test

	Prostate-specific antigen concentration (ng/mL)
8 AM	3.1
12 PM	3.3
4 PM	3.7
8 PM	3.2
12 AM	3.0
Mean value	3.3
Standard deviation	0.3

Coefficient of variation = (standard deviation/mean) × 100 % = 0.3/3.3 × 100% = 9.1%

12.4.2.2   Kappa

For binary tests, which can return only two possible values, reliability can be reported as percent agreement or using the kappa statistic. For example, let's say that two physicians evaluate the reliability of the potassium hydroxide test for diagnosing cutaneous fungal infections. Each physician performs the test independently in 20 consecutive patients who present with itchy skin lesions. Their findings are presented in Table 12.12.

Cells a and d represent pairs of tests in which the two observers agree on the result, whereas cells b and c represent pairs that are discordant. A simple way to summarize these findings is to calculate the proportion of tests that agree:

Percent agreement = number of tests that agree / total number of tests × 100%

$$= (5+30) / (5+3+2+30) \times 100\% = 88\%$$

Table 12.12 Reliability of a binary test from two observers

	Observer one	
	--------------	-----------
Observer two	Positive	Negative
Positive	5 (*a*)	3 (*b*)
Negative	2 (*c*)	30 (*d*)

However, some agreement may occur due to chance alone, even for an imprecise test. The Kappa statistic is used to describe test agreement beyond that expected from chance.

$$\text{Kappa} = \left(\text{percent agreement} - \text{chance agreement}\right) / \left(1 - \text{chance agreement}\right)$$

where chance agreement = $(a + b/\text{total}) \times (a + c/\text{total}) + (b + d/\text{total}) \times (c + d/\text{total})$.
    For the example of the potassium hydroxide test:

Percent agreement	= 0.88
Chance agreement	= $(8/40) \times (7/40) + (33/40) \times (32/40) = 0.04 + 0.66 = 0.70$
Kappa	= $(0.88 - 0.70) / (1 - 0.70) = 0.6$

Values of the Kappa statistic range from +1.0, which indicates perfect agreement, to −1.0, which indicates perfect disagreement. A value 0 indicates no agreement beyond that expected from chance. In general, absolute Kappa statistic values >0.6 are considered to represent reasonably good agreement; values 0.2–0.6 are considered to represent intermediate agreement; and values <0.2 are considered to represent poor agreement.

12.5   Defining Cut Points for Continuous Tests

Many screening and diagnostic tests return naturally continuous results, meaning that they can take on a theoretically infinite number of possible values. The results of continuous tests are often classified as "positive" or "negative" based on some predetermined *cutoff value*. For example, expert guidelines have defined a "positive" PSA test by a serum level >4.0 ng/mL and a "negative" test by a level ≤4.0 ng/mL. Each possible cutoff value applied to a continuous test will generate unique sensitivity and specificity values for that test. Table 12.13 presents sensitivity and specificity values for six possible cutoff values used to define a positive PSA test.

    Selecting a relatively low cutoff value to define a positive PSA test would create a highly sensitive test. In other words, most men who have actual prostate cancer would be expected to test positive if the cutoff value to define a postive test is low. On the other hand, choosing a relatively low cutoff value would also yield a test with low specificity, because many men without actual prostate cancer would also test positive. Increasing the cutoff value used to define a positive PSA test will reduce the sensitivity of the test while increasing specificity.

Table 12.13 Selection of cutoff values for the prostate-specific antigen test

Cutoff value (ng/mL)	Definition of a positive test (ng/mL)	Definition of a negative test (ng/mL)	Sensitivity	Specificity
0	>0	0	1.0	0
1.0	>1.0	≤1.0	0.90	0.20
3.0	>3.0	≤3.0	0.80	0.60
4.0	>4.0	≤4.0	0.60	0.75
5.0	>5.0	≤5.0	0.50	0.80
10.0	>10.0	≤10.0	0	1.0

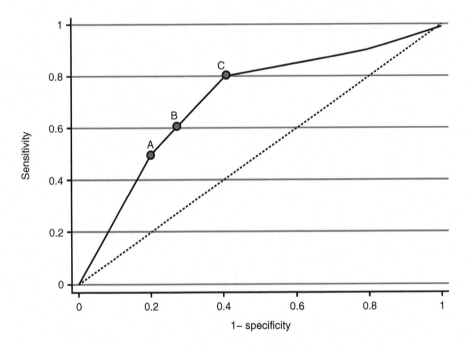

Fig. 12.6 Receiver operating characteristic curve for the PSA test

The trade-off between sensitivity and specificity for all possible cutoff values of a continuous test can be illustrated graphically using a receiver operating characteristic (ROC) curve (Fig. 12.6).

The y-axis of the ROC curve represents the sensitivity of the test, and, by convention, the x-axis represents $1 -$ specificity. The solid line represents the ROC curve for the PSA test, and the dashed diagonal line represents an ROC curve for a hypothetical test that is completely uninformative for detecting prostate cancer. Note that ROC curves typically do not display the actual cutoff values on the graph itself. The data from Table 12.13 are needed to determine the specific PSA cutoff values that were used to construct this ROC curve. For example, point A on the curve has a sensitivity of 0.5 and specificity of $(1 - 0.2) = 0.8$, which correspond to a PSA cutoff value of 5.0 ng/mL, based on Table 12.13.

To gain familiarity with ROC curves, consider the appearance of such a curve for a completely uninformative test. For example, consider the use of height as a test for prostate cancer. The selection of an extremely low cutoff value for height to define a positive test, such as 60 inches, would have nearly 100% sensitivity, because most men who have actual prostate cancer are taller than 60 inches. However, a cutoff value of 60 inches would also have close to 0% specificity, because nearly all men without actual prostate cancer would also test positive. The 100% sensitivity and 0% specificity values are located at the upper right-hand corner of the ROC curve. Gradually raising the cutoff value for height used to define a positive test will monotonically trade off sensitivity at the expense of specificity, because height is irrelevant to the diagnosis of prostate cancer. In other words, the dashed diagonal line on the ROC curve represents the sensitivity and specificity values expected from chance alone.

In contrast, the PSA test, depicted by the solid line, demonstrates some ability to correctly discriminate between men with and without prostate cancer, because sensitivity increases without concomitant loss of specificity across the range of cutoff values. An ROC curve for a theoretically perfect test, which would correctly classify all cases of a disease, would begin at the origin, rise straight up to a sensitivity of 1.0, and then move horizontally across the top of the graph.

ROC curves can be helpful for selecting cutoff values for continuous tests by presenting the sensitivity and specificity for all possible cutoff values of the test. As an initial starting point, the point on ROC curve that lies closest to upper left-hand corner represents the mathematically optimal tradeoff between sensitivity and specificity. However, the ideal cutoff value for a test depends not only on sensitivity and specificity but also on the prevalence of the disease in the tested population, the natural history of the disease if left untreated, the diagnostic procedures that follow a positive test, and the impact of treatment on people who test positive. For the PSA test, a cutoff value of 4.0 ng/mL (point B) represents a reasonable balance between sensitivity and specificity. Nonetheless, the relatively low specificity of the test at this cutoff value will lead to many false positives when the test is applied to a population with a low prevalence of prostate cancer. A positive PSA test may prompt referral for prostate biopsy, which is invasive and expensive. Moreover, many prostate cancers detected by biopsy are low grade and of little consequence to long-term outcomes. Selecting a higher cutoff value for the PSA test, such as 5.0 ng/mL, would increase the specificity of the test and reduce the number of false positives, which may be preferred when applying the test to a low-risk population. However, the increase in specificity would be offset by a decrease in sensitivity, which would result in missing more cancers. The unexceptional ability of the PSA test to correctly identify prostate cancers and the modest mortality benefit associated with treating screen-identified men with these cancers has reduced enthusiasm for testing.

ROC curves can also be used to evaluate the overall predictive capability of a continuous test across all possible cutoff values. The predictive capacity is reported by the *C-statistic*, which is the area under the ROC curve. C-statistic values range from 100% for a perfect test to 50% for a test that is no better than chance (the area under the dashed diagonal line is 50% of the graph area). C-statistic values >0.8 indicate generally good overall predictive capacity.

The C-statistic can also be used to compare predictive capabilities among several different tests for the same disease. For example, ROC curves for the standard and high sensitivity troponin tests, which are used to diagnose myocardial infarction, can be superimposed on the same graph and their respective C-statistics compared to assess overall test validity across the full range of cutoff values.

12.6 Types of Biases in Screening Studies

Observational studies that compare outcomes of people who undergo screening versus those who do not undergo such procedures can provide important information for inferring the impact of screening programs. Nonetheless, observational studies of screening require careful interpretation to ensure that bias has not occurred.

12.6.1 Confounding (Referral Bias)

Observational studies that examine screening programs are subject to confounding by the characteristics that motivate referral for testing. On one hand, screened individuals may be relatively healthy, due to a greater interest in their personal health or the receipt of care from highly attentive providers. On the other hand, people may be referred for testing based on their risk factors for a disease, such as a family history or high-risk behaviors. Referral bias describes confounding that may occur when differences in the characteristics of screened versus unscreened individuals distort the observed association between receipt of a screening test and the study outcomes. For example, an observational study reported that women who received a specialized MRI procedure to screen for breast cancer had improved survival from the disease compared to women who did not undergo this procedure. Referral bias may have occurred if some or all of this observed survival benefit was due to differences in the characteristics of women who underwent MRI screening versus those who did not.

Approaches to control for confounding include randomization, restriction, stratification, matching, and regression (Chap. 10). For nonrandomized studies, careful measurement and control of characteristics that may differ between screened and unscreened individuals are important for obtaining valid results.

12.6.2 Lead Time Bias

A more complex problem may arise in observational studies that compare survival from the time of diagnosis among persons whose disease was or was not detected by screening.

Example 12.5 A hypothetical lung cancer detection program performs annual chest X-ray screening in 5000 asymptomatic lifelong smokers. The program identifies 50 occult lung cancers; all are subsequently treated with appropriate radiation and chemotherapy regimens. To evaluate the effectiveness of the screening program, researchers compare the mortality rate of 50 people whose lung cancers were detected by the screening program to that of a matched group of lung cancer patients whose cancers are identified at the time of clinical presentation. The study finds lower rates of death among the patients whose cancers were detected by X-ray screening, prompting the researchers to conclude that the screening program prolongs survival.

First, the possibility of referral bias should be considered by comparing the characteristics of patients whose cancer was detected by X-ray screening to those whose cancer was identified clinically. However, even if these groups had comparable characteristics, the observed benefit from screening likely derived from artificial differences in survival time.

For patients whose lung cancer was detected by screening, follow-up time began during the preclinical phase of the disease, when the cancer was detected by chest X-ray. In contrast, for unscreened patients whose cancer was detected when it produced recognizable signs and/or symptoms, follow-up time began later in the natural course of the disease, shown in Fig. 12.7.

Even if earlier treatment of lung cancer was no better than the treatment of late cancer, the X-ray screening program would appear to provide survival benefit due to preferential addition of follow-up time to the screened group.

Lead time bias can be addressed by conducting randomized trials of screening programs, in which participants are assigned to different screening procedures or no

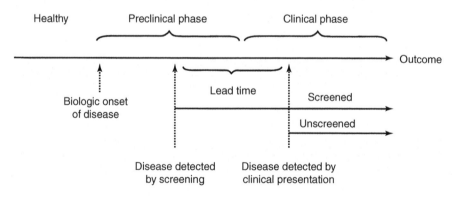

Fig. 12.7 Lead time bias in studies of screening

Method of cancer detection	Number of people	Number of deaths	Follow-up time (years)	Mortality rate (per 1000 person-years)
Chest X-ray screening	50	27	3850 (includes lead time)	7.0
Clinical presentation	50	27	2420	11.6

such screening. Clinical trials would initiate follow-up at the time of randomization, preventing the possibility of systematic inflation of risk time in one of the groups. Observational studies that compare outcomes of screened versus unscreened individuals can attempt to estimate the amount of lead time that is present in their study and correct for this discrepancy in the analyses. Alternatively, observational studies can be performed in which the timing of the diagnosis is not considered, such as in case-control studies.

12.6.3 Length Bias Sampling

A second problem may arise in studies that compare survival from the time of diagnosis among people whose disease was detected by screening versus people whose disease was detected at the time of clinical presentation. Many diseases vary in their rate of progression. For example, some lung cancers follow a rapidly progressive course, with accelerated growth and a tendency toward metastasis, whereas other lung cancers grow relatively more slowly. The administration of a screening test at a single point in time will preferentially favor identification of the slowest progressing variants of a particular disease.

Consider five people who will develop lung cancer at some point during their life span, shown in Fig. 12.8. The time between biologic onset and clinical disease (preclinical phase) varies to some degree among these cancers. The administration of a chest X-ray to screen for lung cancer at a single point in time will preferentially identify cancers that have the longest preclinical phase or slowest growth. Consequently, the disease variants detected by screening programs tend to be less aggressive than those identified by clinical presentation.

12.7 Levels of Prevention

Treatments to prevent the onset or sequelae of disease are categorized into *levels of prevention*.

12.7.1 Primary Prevention

Primary prevention describes the administration of treatments intended to prevent the occurrence of a disease. A classic example of a primary prevention is the provision of immunizations to prevent infectious diseases, such as influenza and measles. Primary preventions may target healthy people, such as for immunizations, or people with disease risk factors, such as referring smokers to smoking cessation programs to prevent the development of peripheral arterial disease.

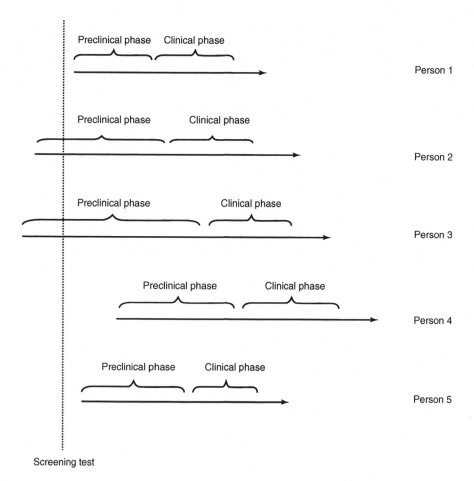

Screening test

Fig. 12.8 Length bias sampling in studies of screening

12.7.2   Secondary Prevention

Secondary prevention describes the provision of treatments that target subclinical disease detected by screening. Examples of secondary prevention include the removal of precancerous polyps identified by colonoscopy and the administration of antiresorptive medications to prevent hip fracture among women who have osteoporosis detected by bone mineral density testing.

12.7.3   Tertiary Prevention

Tertiary prevention describes treatments that target the complications of an existing disease, which include conditions detected by clinical presentation and those confirmed by diagnostic testing. Examples of tertiary prevention include the administration of an angiotensin receptor blocker to prevent kidney disease complications in the setting of diabetes and provision of a beta blocker to reduce the risk of death after a myocardial infarction.

12.8   Association Is Not Sufficient for Prediction

Many risk factors that are associated with disease, including characteristics that may cause the disease, often function poorly as screening or diagnostic tests. Consider a hypothetical new circulating factor that is suspected to play a role in the development of type II diabetes. The factor is released by adipocytes and impairs glucose uptake in skeletal muscle. Researchers measure circulating levels of the new factor in a study of 1000 men and women who do not have clinical diabetes at the start of the study but are at increased risk for developing the disease based on a body mass index >30 kg/m^2 and a family history of diabetes.

Table 12.14 presents the association of the new circulating factor with the incidence of diabetes over 5 years of follow-up.

The relative risk of 3.0 indicates a strong association between the new circulating factor and diabetes outcomes. Given the observational study design, it is possible that people who have detectable levels of the circulating factor differed from those who do not have this factor, potentially confounding the observed association. Adjustment for some diabetes risk factors, such as age, waist circumference, and usual physical activity levels, would help address the possibility of confounding. These results were observed in a high-risk population; replication in other populations would address external validity.

The strong observed association, presence of the circulating factor prior to the occurrence of diabetes (temporality), and plausibility based on the suspected biological effects of the new factor on skeletal muscle suggest a possible causal role in the development of type II diabetes. Evidence of a dose-dependent relationship, which would be indicated by associations of higher levels of the new factor with a progressively greater incidence of type II diabetes, would strengthen the case for a causal relationship. These results are important for advancing understanding of the causes of type II diabetes and motivating follow-up studies that could suggest potential new targets for future treatments.

Consider the identical study data for evaluating the new circulating factor as a possible screening test for diabetes, in which a "positive test" is defined by the presence of detectable levels of the circulating factor, shown in Table 12.15.

Table 12.14 Association of circulating factor with incident type II diabetes

	Incident diabetes		
Circulating factor	Yes	No	Total
Present	100	150	250
Absent	100	650	750

Unadjusted relative risk = (100/250)/(100/750) = 3.0

The circulating factor has only modest utility for correctly classifying cases of incident type II diabetes in this study population. The low positive predictive value indicates that the test will generate numerous false-positive results. The frequency of false positives would be even greater if the test were applied to a more general population with a lower incidence of diabetes. Moreover, a nontrivial number of people with a negative test still develop type II diabetes during follow-up (false negatives). The substantial overlap in the status of the circulating factor between people who develop or do not develop diabetes limits the utility of the factor as a screening test.

In general, the size of an association between a characteristic and disease must be extremely large for that characteristic to perform well as a screening or diagnostic test [2]. Relative risks greater than 10 typically represent a reasonable starting point. For example, when judged using the analytic approach of an association study, a positive mammogram is associated with an approximate 20-fold greater risk of breast cancer, compared with a negative mammogram, yet mammography remains an imperfect screening test (Table 12.16).

Table 12.15 Prediction of type II diabetes outcomes by circulating factor

Circulating factor	Incident cardiovascular disease		Total
	Yes	No	
Present (positive test)	100	150	250
Absent (negative test)	100	650	750

Sensitivity = 100/200 = 0.50
Specificity = 650/800 = 0.81
Positive predictive value = 100/250 = 0.40
Negative predictive value = 650/750 = 0.87

Table 12.16 Likelihood ratios for common clinical conditions [3]

Condition	Diagnostic test	LR+	LR−
Abdominal abscess	Abdominal ultrasound	19.2	0.04
Acute cerebral hemorrhage	Head computed tomography	23.8	0.05
Acute cholecystitis	Abdominal ultrasound	23.8	0.05
Acute myocardial infarction	Cardiac enzymes	32.3	0.03
Aortic stenosis	Echocardiogram	2.6	0.14
Brain tumor	Head computed tomography	31.7	0.05
Breast cancer	Mammogram	8.7	0.14
Breast cancer	Clinical breast exam	3.8	0.69
Clostridium difficile colitis	Clostridium difficile toxin assay	19.6	0.02
Coronary artery disease	Exercise ECG – 1 mm depression	3.5	0.45
Coronary artery disease – women	Exercise echocardiogram	4.29	0.18
Coronary artery disease – women	Exercise thallium test	2.87	0.36
Coronary artery disease – women	Exercise treadmill test	2.25	0.55
Carotid atherosclerosis	Duplex ultrasound	9	0.11
Common duct stone	Abdominal ultrasound	3.8	0.76
COPD (in middle-aged patients)	Forced expiratory volume <80%	2.7	0.81
Endocarditis	Erythrocyte sedimentation rate >20	23	0.07
Endocarditis	Echocardiogram	9.3	0.66
Iron deficiency anemia	Serum transferrin <16.6% saturation	3.2	0.06
Hematuria	Urine dipstick	6.4	0.06
Lung cancer	Chest X-ray	15	0.42
Left ventricular hypertrophy	Echocardiogram	18.4	0.08
Myocardial infarction	Electrocardiogram, single	28.5	0.44
Myocardial infarction	Electrocardiogram, serial	68	0.32
Osteomyelitis	Plain film – bone	5.6	0.55
Acute pancreatitis	Serum amylase	47.5	0.05
Acute pancreatitis	Serum lipase	87	0.13
Renal artery stenosis	Renal scan	4.1	0.28
Systemic lupus	Antinuclear antibodies	4.5	0.125
Systemic lupus	Anti-DNA antibodies >1:80	73	0.27
Chronic subdural hematoma	Head computed tomography	15.5	0.07
Temporal arteritis	Erythrocyte sedimentation rate >20	24.8	0.01
Ureteral obstruction	Abdominal ultrasound	9.8	0.02

LR+ indicates positive likelihood ratio; LR− indicates negative likelihood ratio

References

1. Cohen JD, Li L, Wang Y, et al. Detection and localization of surgically resectable cancers with a multi-analyte blood test. Science. 2018;359:eaar3247.
2. Ware JH. The limitations of risk factors as prognostic tools. N Engl J Med. 2006;355(25):2615–7.
3. Data obtained from http://www.med.unc.edu/medicine/edursrc/lrdis.htm.

Part II
Biostatistics

Chapter 13
Summary Measures in Statistics

Summary of Learning Points

13.1 Three types of variables are commonly encountered in clinical research studies.

    13.1.1 Continuous variables can assume an infinite number of possible values.

    13.1.2 Binary variables can assume only two possible values.

    13.1.3 Categorical variables can assume only a few possible values.

13.2 Univariate statistics are summary measures that pertain to a single variable.

    13.2.1 A histogram plots the observed values of a variable on the x-axis versus the relative frequency of these values on the y-axis.

    13.2.2 The mean is a measure of the center of the data that is sensitive to outlying values.

    13.2.3 The median refers to the value within a distribution for which exactly half of the data fall above this value and half fall below it.

    13.2.4 Disagreement between the mean and median values suggests a skewed distribution.

    13.2.5 The interquartile range is defined as the 25th and 75th quantiles of a distribution.

13.3 Some techniques to describe the joint distribution of two study variables include tabulation across categories, scatter plots, correlation, and quantile-continuous plots.

    13.3.1 Correlation coefficients are used to describe the amount of agreement between two continuous variables.

13.1 Types of Variables

Most variables used in clinical research studies can be described as belonging to one of three categories: continuous, categorical, or binary.

© Springer Nature Switzerland AG 2019
B. Kestenbaum, *Epidemiology and Biostatistics*,
https://doi.org/10.1007/978-3-319-96644-1_13

Continuous variables can take on an infinite number of possible values theoretically arising from anywhere along a (perhaps truncated) number line. Examples of continuous variables include body temperature, serum cholesterol levels, and left ventricular mass. Many continuous variables in clinical research studies can assume only positive values, such as weight and blood pressure, because negative values for these variables are scientifically impossible.

Binary variables can take on only two possible values, for example, biological sex. Binary variables are often used as *indicator variables*, which assume the value of 1 if a specific characteristic or disease is present and 0 if it is not. For example, aspirin use may be represented by an indicator variable that will be equal to 1 if a study participant is using aspirin and 0 if they are not. Binary variables are also called *dichotomous* variables.

Categorical variables can take on only a few possible values, for example, race or cancer stage. Categorical variables can be further classified as *ordered* when the possible responses correspond to a hierarchical scale. For example, the severity of chronic kidney disease is graded on a scale from 1 (mild) to 5 (most severe). Categorical variables with no ordered distinction among the possible responses are classified as *nominal*. Examples of nominal categorical variables include marital status (never married, married, widowed, or divorced) and employment (full-time work, part-time work, unemployed, or retired).

Continuous variables can be transformed into categorical or binary variables for the purpose of analysis. For example, body mass index, a naturally continuous variable, can be transformed into an ordered categorical variable with clinically accepted responses of "normal" (<25 kg/m^2), "overweight" (25-30 kg/m^2), and "obese" (>30 kg/m^2). If accepted scientific or clinical categories have not been previously described, then continuous variables may be transformed into groups containing equal numbers of people, such as quartiles (four equally sized groups) or quintiles (five equally sized groups).

13.2   Univariate Statistics

13.2.1   Histograms

Clinical research studies typically evaluate too many subjects to list *all* of the observed values for any particular variable. For example, it would be impractical to list the systolic blood pressures of every person in most research studies. Instead, a condensed description of study variables is desired for presentation. A *summary measure* is a compact description of one or more study variables that conveys information about the distribution of these variables quickly. Summary measures pertaining to a single variable are called *univariate statistics*.

One example of a summary measure is a *histogram*, which plots the observed values of a variable on the *x*-axis versus the relative frequency of these values on the *y*-axis. For example, systolic blood pressure data of more than 6000 participants in a community-based cohort study are described by the histogram in Fig. 13.1, which conveys a sense of how the blood pressure values are distributed in the study population.

The *y*-value represents the frequency (%) of each systolic blood pressure value in the study. The arrow in the figure indicates that about 4% of the systolic blood pressures are between 150 and 155 mmHg. The tallest bar represents the most commonly occurring systolic blood pressure value of 115 mmHg. The histogram demonstrates that "typical" systolic pressures in this study are between 100 and 150 mmHg, with occasional extreme values greater than 200 mmHg.

Figure 13.2 presents a second histogram describing serum levels of C-reactive protein (CRP), an inflammatory biomarker, in this same 6000-person study.

The CRP histogram has a very different shape than that of systolic blood pressure. Most participants in the study have very low CRP levels; in fact, more than 30% of participants have a value close to 0 mg/L. However, a decreasingly small number of people have progressively higher levels of CRP.

The histogram for systolic blood pressure would be considered to represent an approximately "normal" distribution, because the data appear to be shaped roughly like a bell-shaped curve. Close inspection of the histogram for blood pressure reveals a small nonsymmetric bump on the right side that distracts from an otherwise clean, bell-shaped appearance. A more descriptive categorization of the blood pressure

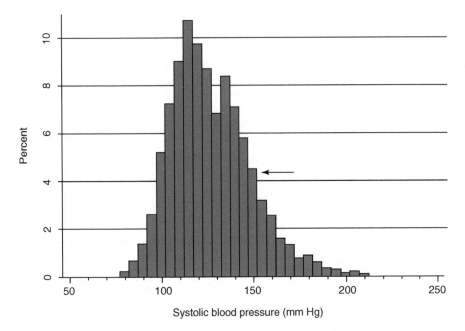

Fig. 13.1 Histogram of systolic blood pressure values in a community-based study. Each bar on the *x*-axis is 5 mmHg wide

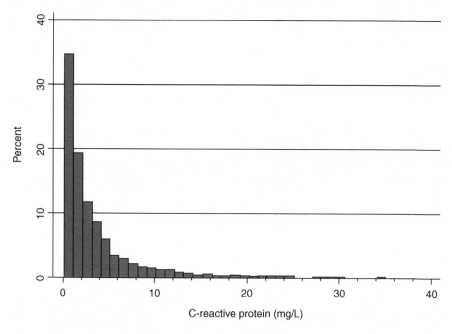

Fig. 13.2 Histogram of C-reactive protein values

data would be "normal appearing with some rightward skew" to describe the more drawn out tail on the right side of the histogram. The term *skew* refers to the degree of asymmetry in a distribution. In contrast, the CRP histogram demonstrates a variable that is clearly *not* normally distributed, with a large amount of rightward skew.

13.2.2 Measures of Location and Spread

In addition to describing the general shape of a distribution, histograms also provide graphical information regarding "typical" values for a particular variable and the range of observed values for that variable. Formally, estimates of the "typical" value in a distribution are termed *measures of location*, and estimates of how far apart the data are located from this typical value are termed *measures of spread*.

The most common measure of location is the arithmetic *mean*. Statistically, the mean is the expected value of a variable, and in many circumstances, the mean will be a reasonable description of the middle of the data. The mean is calculated by summing all of the observed values of a variable and then dividing by the total number of observations.

$$\text{Mean} = \frac{\sum x_i}{N}$$

Where x_i refers to each value in a distribution and N refers to the number of observations in that distribution. The most common measure of spread is the *standard deviation*. Distributions with a high standard deviation will be very spread out, whereas distributions with a low standard deviation will be tightly grouped. The standard deviation is calculated as the square root of the variance.

$$\text{Variance} = \frac{\Sigma(\mu - x_i)^2}{N} \quad \text{Standard deviation} = \sqrt{(\text{variance})}$$

where μ represents the mean value.

Calculation of the variance requires going through each value in a distribution, computing the distance between that value and the mean value, squaring that distance, and then dividing the sum of the squared distances by the total number of observations. Thankfully, this is accomplished by a keystroke on a computer.

Research studies often present the mean value of a continuous variable along with its standard deviation. For example, the mean systolic blood pressure in the 6000-person cohort study is 126.6 mmHg, and the standard deviation is 21.5 mmHg. If a variable is normally distributed, then 67% of the values will fall within one standard deviation of the mean value, and 95% of values will fall within two standard deviations of the mean. Since the histogram for systolic blood pressure reveals a roughly normal-appearing distribution, we can expect that approximately 95% of study participants will have a systolic blood pressure within two standard deviations of the mean value of 126.6 mmHg, or $126.6 \pm (21.5 \times 2) = (83.6, 169.6)$ mmHg, as shown in Fig. 13.3.

The arithmetic mean is fairly sensitive to extreme values of a distribution. For example, the mean income for a particular town may not reflect the "typical" income for that town if the majority of residents earn between \$20,000 and \$120,000, but there is also one billionaire. The mean CRP value in the 6000-person cohort study is 3.8 mg/L; however, inspection of the histogram in Fig. 13.2 reveals that 3.8 mg/L is *not* a typical CRP value for this population. The mean CRP value is highly influenced by the few individuals who have extremely high CRP levels. Better options for describing typical values for highly skewed distributions are the *median* and the *geometric mean*, which are less sensitive to extreme values.

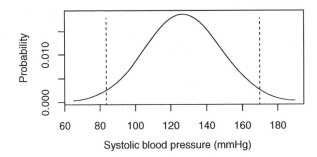

Fig. 13.3 Normal distribution; 95% of data is within two standard deviations of the mean

The geometric mean is calculated by taking the arithmetic mean of log-transformed data and then converting back to the original scale by exponentiation (taking the antilog). In symbols:

$$\text{Geometric mean} = \exp\left[\frac{\sum \ln(x_i)}{N}\right]$$

where ln represents the natural log.

The geometric mean of the CRP data is 1.9 mg/L. This value is less influenced by outlying values that reside far from most of the other values.

13.2.3 Quantiles

Another common method to describe the distribution of a variable is *quantiles* or *percentiles*. Quantiles describe specific values within a distribution that divide the data into groups. For example, 90% of participants in the 6,000-person cohort study have a CRP level less than 9.0 mg/L. Therefore, the 90th percentile for the CRP distribution is 9.0 mg/L. The 50th quantile, also called the *median*, refers to the value within a distribution for which exactly half of the data fall above this value and half fall below it. The median CRP level is 1.9 mg/L, meaning that half of the participants have a CRP level that is less than 1.9 mg/L and half have a level that is greater than 1.9 mg/L. The 25th and 75th quantiles of a distribution are also called the *interquartile range*.

In this example, the mean CRP value of 3.8 mg/L differs notably from the median value of 1.9 mg/L. Disagreement between the mean and median values within a distribution suggests that the variable is *not* normally distributed but is instead skewed.

Continuous variables are sometimes converted into categorical variables using quantiles. For example, continuous values of CRP could be divided into three, four, or five groups containing equal numbers of people, known as tertiles, quartiles, and quintiles, respectively. The creation of quantiles facilitates presentation of the data, shown in Table 13.1.

Table 13.1 Quartiles of serum CRP levels in a community-based study

	CRP level (mg/L)			
	Quartile 1	Quartile 2	Quartile 3	Quartile 4
	0.1–0.7 mg/L	0.8–1.8 mg/L	1.9–4.2 mg/L	4.2–27 mg/L
Number of participants	1500	1500	1500	1500
Age (years)	61 ± 11	63 ± 11	63 ± 10	61 ± 10
Systolic blood pressure (mmHg)	123 ± 22	126 ± 21	129 ± 22	129 ± 21
Waist circumference (cm)	91 ± 12	96 ± 12	101 ± 14	105 ± 15

All values in the table are expressed as mean ± standard deviation

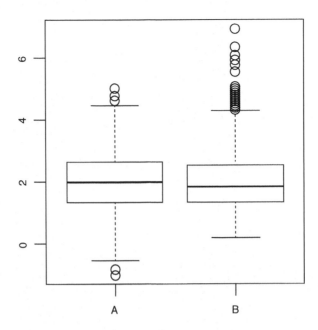

Fig. 13.4 Box plots for two distributions with the same mean and standard deviation

Quantiles can be displayed graphically using *box plots*, which contain three main data elements: (1) a shaded region representing the 25th and 75th quantiles (*interquartile range*), (2) a horizontal bar representing the median value, and (3) "whiskers" that typically extend to 1.5 times the 25th and 75th quantiles or to the minimum and maximum observation, whichever is less extreme. Additional extreme observations are displayed in box plots as open circles beyond the whiskers. Figure 13.4 presents box plots for the distributions of two hypothetical variables A and B that have the same mean and standard deviation.

The box plots indicate that variable B has a slightly lower median value and a greater number of outlier observations compared with variable A. Note that the mean and standard deviation are not shown on the box plots.

13.2.4 Univariate Statistics for Binary Data

For binary data, the arithmetic mean is exactly equal to the proportion of people who have a characteristic of interest. For example, aspirin use may be represented by a binary variable that assumes a value of 1 if a person uses aspirin or 0 if they do not. A mean value of 0.25 for the aspirin use variable would indicate that 25% of that population uses aspirin.

The standard deviation of binary data is calculated directly from known mathematical properties. For a binary variable with a mean value of p:

$$\text{Standard deviation} = \sqrt{\left[p \times (1 - p) \right]}$$

The standard deviation of the aspirin use variable would be $\sqrt{[0.25 \times (1-0.25)]} = 0.43$.

For categorical data, the mean value is rarely scientifically meaningful. For such data, the primary interest is in the percentage of people within each classification.

13.3   Bivariate Statistics

13.3.1   Tabulation Across Categories

Bivariate descriptive statistics are used to describe the joint relationship between two variables of interest. For binary or categorical variables, joint distributions with other study variables can be presented in tabular form. Consider a cohort study that examines the association of aspirin use with the incidence of stroke. The binary aspirin use variable can be tabulated in relation to the baseline characteristics of the study participants, shown in Table 13.2.

The baseline characteristics table presents the joint distribution of the aspirin use variable with other continuous study variables (age, systolic blood pressure, weight) and binary variables (sex, current smoking, diabetes). Note that binary variables are typically presented as mean (number of people) rather than mean (standard deviation), because the standard deviation of a binary variable is simply calculated from the mean value as $\sqrt{[p \times (1 - p)]}$.

13.3.2   Correlation

The comparison of two continuous variables can be assessed graphically using *scatter plots*. Figure 13.5 presents three scatter plots describing the association of weight with height, age, and HDL-cholesterol levels.

Scatter plots present a subjective description of the joint distribution between two continuous variables, but do not provide an objective measure of the strength of

Table 13.2 Baseline characteristics in a cohort study of aspirin use and stroke

	Aspirin use ($N = 1000$)	No aspirin use ($N = 1500$)
Age (years)	65.0 ± 10.2	65.5 ± 9.6
Systolic blood pressure (mmHg)	132.3 ± 21.3	125.4 ± 21.4
Weight (pounds)	179.0 ± 36.8	171.2 ± 38.7
Female	512 (51.2)	809 (53.9)
Current smoking	109 (10.9)	245 (16.3)
Diabetes	141 (14.1)	197 (13.1)

All values expressed as mean ± standard deviation or number of participants (percent)

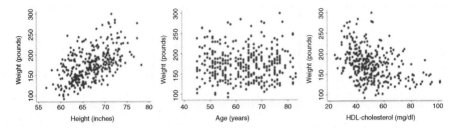

Fig. 13.5 Scatter plots depicting associations between two continuous variables

the association. *Correlation* is an objective summary measure used to describe the joint distribution of two continuous variables by measuring the tendency of larger values of one variable to match up with larger values of a second variable. A correlation coefficient of +1.0 describes perfect positive agreement between two variables, such that higher values of the first variable are always linked with higher values of the second variable. A correlation coefficient of −1.0 describes perfect negative agreement, such that higher values of the first variable are always linked with lower values of the second variable. A correlation coefficient of 0 indicates no agreement between the two variables. The correlation coefficient for the scatter plot relating weight and height in Fig. 13.5 is +0.54, indicating some positive agreement between these characteristics. The correlation coefficient for weight and age is +0.01, indicating no agreement, and the correlation coefficient for weight and HDL-C cholesterol levels is –0.37, indicating some negative agreement.

13.3.3 Quantile-Continuous Variable Plots

Continuous variables may also be plotted as a function of quantiles of a second variable. A classic example is a pediatric growth chart, shown in Fig. 13.6, for boys.

The growth chart displays different quantiles for weight (5th, 25th, 50th, 75th, and 95th quantiles), plotted on the *y*-axis, as a function of age, plotted on the *x*-axis. This chart demonstrates that the median weight of a 10-year-old boy is about 75 pounds, meaning that half of 10-year-old boys would be expected to have a weight below 75 pounds and half would be expected to have a weight above this value. The interquartile range for the weight of 10-year-old boys is 65–95 pounds, describing the middle 50% of the data. A weight below 58 pounds is expected in less than 5% of 10-year-old boys.

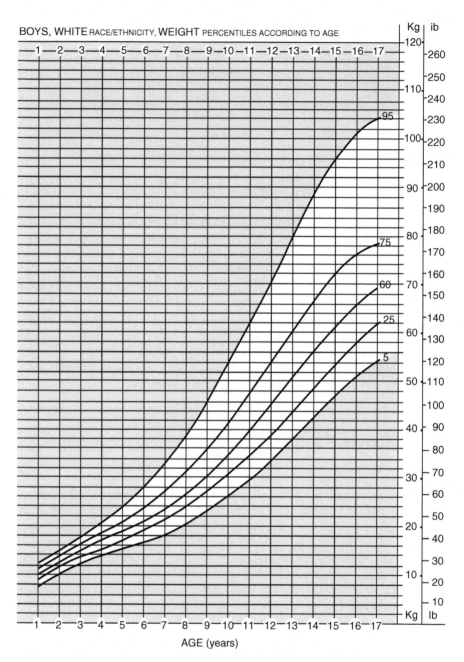

Fig. 13.6 Example of quantile-continuous plot: pediatric growth chart for boys

Chapter 14
Introduction to Statistical Inference

Summary of Learning Points

14.1 A population refers to a theoretically infinite group of people who fit some particular description. A sample is a subset of a given population, often selected at random.

14.2 External validity describes whether a given population is clinically or scientifically relevant.

14.3 Statistical inference relates findings obtained from a sample to those in the population.

    14.3.1 A larger sample size and smaller variance increase the likelihood that results obtained from a sample will accurately reflect those in the population.

14.4 If a study is repeated indefinitely, and a 95% confidence interval constructed for each experimental result, then 95% of these intervals will contain the true population value.

14.5 Given a null hypothesis about the underlying population, the *p*-value is the probability of observing the sample result, or a more extreme result, due to sampling variation alone.

14.1 Definition of a Population and a Sample

A *population* refers to all people in the world (or universe) who fit some particular description. A *sample* represents a subset of a given population, often selected at random, and is typically often a small fraction of the population. By definiation, a sample is always completely contained within a given population.

Example 14.1 A cohort study examines the association of aspirin use with incident stroke among 2500 middle-aged men with no previous history of stroke. Researchers determine the use versus nonuse of aspirin at the start of the study and then follow participants over 10 years to ascertain new occurrences of stroke.

© Springer Nature Switzerland AG 2019
B. Kestenbaum, *Epidemiology and Biostatistics*,
https://doi.org/10.1007/978-3-319-96644-1_14

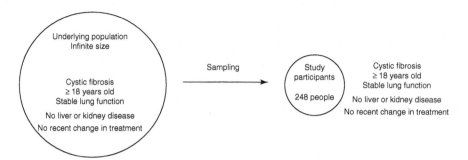

Fig. 14.1 Underlying population and sample in clinical trial of new cystic fibrosis treatment

In this example, the *population* in question would be *all* stroke-free middle-aged men in the world. The 2,500 participants in this particular study (unfortunately referred to as the "study population" even though they are *not* a population) are just one of many possible samples that could be drawn from the population of interest.

Example 14.2 Cystic fibrosis is a progressive disease caused by mutations in the cystic fibrosis transmembrane conductance regulator (CFTR) gene. A randomized clinical trial tested a novel therapy that potentiates activity of the CFTR protein [1]. The trial recruited 248 patients who had a definitive diagnosis of cystic fibrosis, were at least 12 years old, and had stable lung function at the time of enrollment. Exclusion criteria included kidney or liver disease or recent changes in cystic fibrosis treatments.

In this example, the *population* in question would be all people who have a definitive diagnosis of cystic fibrosis and meet these trial eligibility criteria. The 248 participants who were enrolled in the trial represent one of many possible samples that could be selected from the underlying population.

From the definition of a population, human research studies rarely, if ever, evaluate entire populations. However, researchers would like to *infer* whether the results obtained in a particular study are reflective of findings that would be obtained among all similar people. If the new cystic fibrosis treatment is found to slow disease progression among the 248 trial participants, then the researchers would like to infer whether similar effects can be expected in the larger underlying population from which these participants were selected. The impact of research studies would be greatly diminished if the results applied to only the specific people in a study. Figure 14.1 illustrates the underlying population and sample in the cystic fibrosis trial.

14.2 External Validity

External validity is a subjective, *not mathematical*, term that describes whether an underlying population is clinically or scientifically relevant. Consider the eligibility criteria for the cystic fibrosis trial: a definitive diagnosis of the disease, age 12 years and older, stable lung function, no kidney or liver disease, and no recent changes in cystic fibrosis treatment. The role of statistical inference is to relate the results obtained from the 248 participants in the trial to the underlying population of comparable cystic fibrosis patients who meet all of these entry criteria. Whether the trial results are applicable to more general groups of cystic fibrosis patients, who often have at least one of these exclusions, is a question of external validity. Common sense, clinical, and scientific knowledge, *not* statistics, are used to decide whether the underlying population is important and potentially applicable to clinical practice.

14.3 Statistical Inference

Samples selected at random from an underlying population (random sample) may not accurately reflect the qualities of that population simply due to chance. Consider a hypothetical statistics examination for a class of 200 students in which the average score is 90%. Selecting a random sample of 10 students and computing the average score may yield a mean value of 82%. Selecting a second random sample of 10 students and computing the average score may yield a mean value of 97%. Only by sampling the entire population of 200 students would we be guaranteed to find the true mean class score of 90%.

However, definitive information about a characteristic in the underlying population is typically unknown, because studies rarely evaluate entire populations. Inferential statistics uses mathematical properties to estimate characteristics in a population based on the results obtained from a sample of that population. For the example of the statistics exam, researchers would not know that the true average class score was 90% but would use the results obtained from a sample of students to make an *inference* about the mean score in the entire class.

Two characteristics that influence how closely the results obtained from a sample of people will reflect those in the underlying population are *sample size* and *variance*. Sample size is intuitive – larger samples will be more representative of the underlying population from which these samples are drawn, yielding findings that are more likely to be comparable to those in the population. The average statistics exam score obtained from a sample of 100 students is more likely to be similar to the true mean score of 90% than the average score obtained from a sample of only 10 students.

A smaller amount of variance, or spread, in a characteristic will also increase the likelihood that a sample will contain a representative value of a characteristic. If scores on the statistics examination ranged from 85% to 95% among the entire class, then the mean value obtained from a random sample of students would likely be close to 90%. On the other hand, if the exam scores ranged from 40% to 120% (with extra credit), then there will be a greater probability of selecting an unusual sample with a mean score far from the true class average.

14.4 Confidence Intervals

Confidence intervals report an estimated range of plausible values for a characteristic in the underlying population. These intervals are conceptualized, such that if a particular experiment were repeated an infinite number of times, and a 95%

confidence interval constructed for each experiment, then 95% of these intervals will contain the population value of interest.

Consider the following analogy: imagine that an archer is known to be accurate to within 10 cm of the bullseye 95% of the time. Now suppose that you are standing behind the target and don't know the actual location of the bullseye but can see where the archer's arrow strikes the target. One reasonable method to guess the location of the true bullseye is to draw a circle with a radius of 10 cm around the archer's arrow. Since the arrows are known to be within 10 cm of the bullseye 95% of the time, this procedure will include the true bullseye 95% of the time.

For a more practical example, consider a simple experiment to estimate the average weight of the US adult population. Researchers select a random sample of 100 US adults and calculate the mean weight in the sample. Table 14.1 presents results of 20 successive repetitions of this same experiment.

The idea behind confidence intervals is to find some interval that can be placed around each experimental result, such that *95% of all intervals will contain the true result in the population*. For the purposes of this example, we will assume that the mean weight in the entire US population is 160 pounds; however, from a practical standpoint, the population value will nearly always be unknown. A 95% confidence interval for the experiments listed in Table 14.1 would be such an interval that includes the actual mean weight of the US adult population 19/20 or 95% of the time. This interval turns out to be ±11 pounds. Table 14.2 applies this interval to the experimental results.

Table 14.1 Successive experiments to calculate mean weight in samples of 100 US adults

Experiment	Mean weight (pounds)
1	165
2	157
3	149
4	166
5	171
6	148
7	152
8	158
9	155
10	163
11	160
12	157
13	163
14	161
15	149
16	166
17	160
18	152
19	159
20	151

Experiment	Mean weight (pounds)	95% confidence interval (pounds)
1	165	154–176
2	157	146–168
3	149	138–160
4	166	155–177
5	171	160–182
6	148	**137–159**
7	152	141–163
8	158	147–169
9	155	144–166
10	163	152–174
11	160	149–171
12	157	146–168
13	163	152–174
14	161	150–172
15	149	138–160
16	166	155–177
17	160	149–171
18	152	141–163
19	159	148–170
20	151	140–162

Table 14.2 Successive experiments to calculate mean weight with confidence intervals

If an interval of ±11 pounds were placed around the results of each experiment, then 19/20 or 95% of the intervals will contain the true population mean weight of 160 pounds. One of the intervals will exclude the population mean (shown in bold).

Details regarding how to actually compute 95% confidence intervals are beyond the scope of this book. However, *confidence intervals are calculated without knowledge of the true population value using only known mathematical properties of sampling.*

In practice, it is important to *interpret* confidence intervals in the context of a research study. Consider a more practical example of a study to estimate the average weight of the US adult population, in which the experiment is performed only once. Researchers select *one* sample of 100 US adults, calculate the mean weight of the sample, and then use a computer to determine the 95% confidence interval:

$$\text{New experiment}: \text{mean weight} = 155 \text{ pounds}; 95\% \text{confidence interval}$$
$$(144 - 166 \text{ pounds})$$

In this more realistic circumstance, the actual mean weight of the entire US adult population is unknown, because it would be impossible to study the entire US population. Based on the definition of a confidence interval, if this particular experiment were repeated an infinite number of times, and a 95% confidence interval placed around each result, then 95% of these intervals would contain the true mean weight in the US adult population.

Unfortunately, we have no way of knowing whether the 95% confidence interval of 144–166 pounds contains the true mean weight in the US adult population, because the population value is unknown. So, it is technically incorrect to interpret this confidence interval directly as, "there is a 95% chance that the mean weight in the US adult population is between 144 and 166 pounds." We could instead state that we are "95% confident" that this interval contains the true mean weight in the US adult population, because of 95% of all such intervals contain this value.

A less formal but simpler interpretation of the 95% confidence interval would be "we can be '95% confident' that the true mean weight in the US adult population is between 144 and 166 pounds." By design, the term "confident" is mathematically ambiguous. More correctly, we can state that this confidence interval was constructed using a procedure that will contain the true population value in 95% of repeated samples.

Consider the results reported from the study of aspirin use and stroke described in Example 14.1. The study found aspirin use to be associated with a 20% lower incidence of stroke among 2500 middle-aged men who were stroke-free at the start of the study (relative risk = 0.8). The researchers compute a 95% confidence interval for this relative risk of 0.65–0.98.

The relative risk of 0.8 is specific to this particular sample of 2500 stroke-free middle-aged men. The true relative risk of stroke, comparing aspirin use with nonuse, among all similar stroke-free middle-aged men in the population is unknown. However, the 95% confidence interval provides an inference as to the likely range of relative risks in the population. Formally, 95% of all confidence intervals constructed for this experiment will contain the true relative risk of stroke associated with aspirin use in the underlying population of stroke-free middle-aged men. We don't know whether this particular confidence interval of 0.65–0.98 happens to be one that contains the true relative risk, yet 95% of all such intervals do. Applying the less formal interpretation of the confidence interval, "we can be '95% confident' that the relative risk of stroke associated with aspirin use could be as low as 0.65 or as high as 0.98 among all stroke-free middle-aged men in the population." The results obtained from a specific study are used to make an inference about the association of interest in the larger underlying population.

The confidence interval of 0.65–0.98 excludes the value of 1.0, which would be observed if there were no association of aspirin use with stroke. Therefore, we can also be "95% confident" that aspirin use is associated with *some* lower incidence of stroke in the underlying population.

What about the association of aspirin use with stroke among women or older people? These questions pertain to the external validity of the study findings, not statistical inference, because they address the clinical and scientific relevance of the underlying population.

Recall that *sample size* and *variance* impact how closely the results obtained from a sample are likely to reflect those in the underlying population. These factors directly influence the width of the 95% confidence interval. *A larger sample size will generate a narrower confidence interval*, because characteristics obtained from larger samples will be more representative of those in the underlying population. The

Table 14.3 Impact of sample size and sample variance on width of the confidence interval

Sample size (people)	Mean weight (pounds)	Standard deviation (pounds)	95% confidence interval (pounds)
100	158	28	147–169
500	158	28	155–161
500	158	15	156–160

association of aspirin use with stroke obtained from a study of 100,000 stroke-free middle-aged men is more likely to be closer to the true association in the population than that obtained from a study of 2500 such people. The 95% confidence interval for the larger study will be considerably narrower, reflecting greater certainty about the true size of the association in the population.

Lower variance in a characteristic will also yield a narrower confidence interval. Consider the study to determine the mean weight in the US adult population. A study of fixed sample size is more likely to obtain a mean weight close to the population value of 160 pounds if the distribution of weight is tightly grouped around a mean value of 160 pounds. Unfortunately, information regarding the variance of a characteristic in the underlying population is typically unknown. However, the variance calculated from a particular sample can be used to estimate the variance in the population. Smaller variance within a sample, described by a lower standard deviation, will yield a narrower confidence interval.

Table 14.3 presents the results of three hypothetical experiments to determine the mean weight of the US adult population

All three experiments obtain the identical mean weight of 158 pounds. The third experiment, which has the largest sample size and the lowest sample variance, yields the narrowest confidence interval, indicating greater certainty regarding the true mean weight in the population.

What about variance for a binary study outcome such as stroke? Recall from Chap. 13 that the variance of a binary variable with a mean value of p is defined as:

$$\text{Variance} = \left[p \times (1 - p) \right]$$

The highest variance will be obtained for outcomes that have a probability of 0.5, or those that occur in 50% of participants.

14.5 Hypothesis Testing

14.5.1 Construction of Statistical Hypotheses

Hypotheses testing describes a statistical procedure for performing inference testing based on a predefined conjecture about a characteristic of interest in the underlying population. The first step is to construct two mutually exclusive hypotheses about a characteristic in the underlying population before conducting a study.

For the cohort study of aspirin use and stroke, a suitable study hypothesis would be:

Aspirin use is associated with stroke in the population of stroke-free middle-aged men.

The study hypothesis does *not* suppose whether aspirin use is associated with a greater or lesser risk of stroke in the population, only that *some* association is present. Based on the study hypothesis, a mutually exclusive null hypothesis would be:

Aspirin use is not associated with stroke in the population of stroke-free middle-aged men.

The study hypothesis and null hypotheses always pertain to the underlying population. The study hypothesis is also called the *alternative hypothesis*.

14.5.2   P-Values

Following construction of the study and null hypotheses, the study is performed. In this example, researchers recruit 2500 stroke-free middle-aged men, determine aspirin use at the start of the study, and then ascertain new occurrences of stroke over 10 years. The study finds aspirin use to be associated with a 20% lower incidence of stroke (relative risk = 0.8). The researchers compute a *p*-value for this relative risk of 0.03.

The definition of a *p*-value is:

Given a null hypothesis regarding the underlying population, the p-value is the probability of observing a particular sample result, or a more extreme result, due to sampling variation alone.

The *p*-value of 0.03 is interpreted as, "if there is *no association* between aspirin use and stroke among all stroke-free middle-aged men in the population, then the chance of observing a relative risk of 0.8, or a more extreme relative risk, in this particular study is 3%." Stated another way, given no true association between aspirin use and stroke in the underlying population, the chance of selecting an unusual sample of 2500 stroke-free middle-aged men and finding a relative risk of 0.8, or an even more extreme relative risk, due to sample-to-sample variation alone is only 3%. Given such a low probability, it is reasonable to conclude that aspirin use *is* likely to be associated with stroke among all stroke-free middle-aged men. The results obtained from a study of 2500 people were used to make an inference about this association in the population.

To make life more complicated, *p*-values are almost always "two sided," meaning that the phrase "more extreme values" in the *p*-value definition refers to values that are greater than the sample result or less than the opposite result. For the association of aspirin use with stroke, the probability of finding a relative risk of 0.8, or a "more extreme" relative risk, refers to finding relative risks that are ≤ 0.8 *or* relative risks that are $\geq (1.0/0.8) \geq 1.25$, shown in Fig. 14.2.

The procedures used to calculate *p*-values, like those used to calculate confidence intervals, are beyond the scope of this book but are based on known

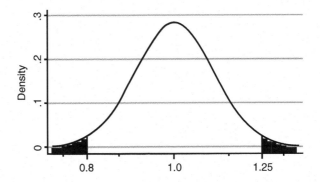

Fig. 14.2 Two-sided probability of observing a relative risk of 0.8 or a more extreme value

mathematical properties of sampling that do not assume any knowledge of the true result in the population. The same characteristics that impact the width of the 95% confidence interval also influence the size of the p-value. Specifically, a larger sample size and a smaller variance will generate a lower p-value.

Note that calculation of the p-value requires construction of a preconceived null hypothesis about the underlying population. Statistical hypothesis testing is set up for proof by contradiction. We first assume that some null hypothesis regarding the population, typically describing no effect or association, is true. We then conduct the experiment in a random sample of people selected from that population and calculate the probability of observing the sample result, or a more extreme result, if the null hypothesis were true. If this probability is small, we then reject the null hypothesis and declare that the alternative (study) hypothesis about the underlying population is likely to be true.

P-values and confidence intervals provide complementary information about a characteristic of interest in the underlying population. For the study of aspirin use and stroke, the p-value of 0.03 implies that *some* association between aspirin use and stroke is likely among all stroke-free middle-aged men in the population. However, the p-value provides no direct information regarding the possible *size* of such an association. The 95% confidence interval of 0.65–0.98 adds that the relative risk of stroke associated with aspirin use is likely to be between 0.65 and 0.98 in the underlying population.

A p-value threshold of 0.05 is often used to judge the validity of experimental results. There is no special meaning to the value of 0.05. This value simply indicates a 5% chance that the null hypothesis is true given the results of the study. Consider a clinical trial that evaluates a novel treatment for glioblastoma, a malignant and highly fatal cancer. Researchers assign 20 patients with glioblastoma to receive either the experimental treatment or the existing standard of care. After 16 weeks, tumor volume is found to decrease by 50% in the experimental group compared with 2% in the standard care group; p-value = 0.10. This p-value can be interpreted as:

Given no effect of the experimental treatment on tumor volume in the population of similar glioblastoma patients, the chance of observing this 50% reduction in tumor volume, or an even greater reduction in tumor volume, is 10%.

There is only a 10% chance of observing this impact of the experimental treatment on tumor volume if the treatment has no true effect on tumor volume in the underlying population of similar glioblastoma patients. Yet, based on a p-value threshold of 0.05, the study findings would be declared as "not statistically significant." It would be premature to conclude from these data that the new treatment has no impact on tumor volume, particularly if the treatment has other promising characteristics, such as a large and clinically important effect on a cancer that is typically unresponsive, an innovative mechanism of action, or a benign side-effect profile. An appropriate next step would be to conduct a larger study of the new treatment to obtain more information regarding the true benefits (and risks) in the underlying population.

Reference

1. Rowe SM, Daines C, Ringshausen FC, et al. Tezacaftor-Ivacaftor in residual-function heterozygotes with cystic fibrosis. N Engl J Med. 2017;377(21):2024–35.

Chapter 15
Hypothesis Tests in Practice

Summary of Learning Points

15.1 Two-sample tests compare a characteristic of interest between two different groups.

    15.1.1 A t-test compares the mean value of a characteristic between two groups.

    15.1.2 A chi-square test compares proportions between two groups.

15.2 Hypothesis testing can lead to errors.

    15.2.1 A type I error occurs when a hypothesis test declares a result to be statistically significant, yet the null hypothesis is true (no actual difference in population).

    15.2.2 A type II error occurs when a hypothesis test declares a result to be statistically nonsignificant, yet the null hypothesis is false (actual difference in population).

15.3 Power is the probability that a study will *not* make a type II error, given a pre-specified assumption about the difference in a characteristic between groups.

    15.3.1 Power is greater for larger sample sizes.

    15.3.2 Power is greater for detecting larger effects or associations in the population.

    15.3.3 Power is greater for outcome measurements that are less variable.

    15.3.4 Power is greater for higher threshold values of statistical significance.

15.1 Two-Sample Hypothesis Tests

A common task in clinical research studies is to test whether a characteristic of interest differs between two different groups in a given population. For example, research studies may wish to compare weight among children who are treated versus not treated with stimulant medications, cognitive function among adults with and without a specific genetic variant, or cardiac ejection fraction among persons with and without thyroid

© Springer Nature Switzerland AG 2019
B. Kestenbaum, *Epidemiology and Biostatistics*,
https://doi.org/10.1007/978-3-319-96644-1_15

disease. Potential differences in these characteristics observed among the people in a particular study may or may not reflect true differences in the underlying population. Two-sample hypothesis tests are statistical procedures that make an inference about the difference in a characteristic between two groups in an underlying population.

15.1.1   T-*Test*

The *t*-test is a statistical test used to compare the *mean value* of a characteristic between two different groups.

Example 15.1 A clinical trial evaluates a new inhaled asthma medication in 100 patients who have an established diagnosis of asthma. Exclusion criteria include current smoking or a recent asthma exacerbation within the previous 6 months. The investigators randomly assign half of the participants to add the new inhaler to their existing asthma medications and the other half to continue with their usual asthma treatments. At the end of the study, participants complete a 6-min walk test, which measures the distance a person can walk on a flat surface over 6 min (lower scores indicate worse performance). The results of the study are presented in Table 15.1.

For the *T*-test, the null hypothesis is that the mean value of the outcome variable is equal between the two groups in the underlying population. The null hypothesis for the above comparison of 6-min walk distances between the two treatment groups would be:

- Six-minute walk distance is *equal* comparing all similar asthma patients who add the new inhaler with all similar asthma patients who receive their existing treatments in the underlying population.

The two-sided study hypothesis (also called the alternative hypothesis) would be:

- Six-minute walk distance is *not equal* comparing all similar asthma patients who add the new inhaler with all similar asthma patients who receive their existing treatments in the underlying population.

Collectively, the null and study hypotheses cover all possible results, such that if one hypothesis is true then the other is necessarily false. The *p*-value from a *t*-test represents the probability of observing the results in a particular sample (study), or

Table 15.1 Comparison of end-of-study 6-min walk distance

	Number of people	Mean end-of-study 6-min walk distance	Standard deviation
Add new inhaler to existing treatment	50	540 m	75 m
Existing treatment alone	50	500 m	75 m

Difference in mean 6-min walk distance = 540–500 = 40 m
T-test: *p*-value = 0.01
95% confidence interval (10 m, 70 m)

more extreme results, if the population means were truly equal (null hypothesis true). The *p*-value of 0.01 from the table is interpreted as:

- If addition of the new inhaler has no true impact on end-of-study 6-min walk distance in the population of all similar asthma patients, then the chance of observing a 40-meter difference, or an even larger difference, in this study of 100 people is 1%.

Such a low probability of the null hypothesis implies that the alternative hypothesis is likely to be true. *The results of this t-test suggest that addition of the new inhaler is likely to have some impact on 6-min walk distance among all similar patients in the underlying population.*

In this example, the underlying population refers to all patients who have an established diagnosis of asthma, are non-smokers, and have no recent asthma exacerbations (the inclusion criteria of the trial). Whether the results of this trial are likely to apply other groups of asthma patients is a question of external validity.

The 95% confidence interval provides complementary information to the *p*-value. The low *p*-value suggests that addition of the new inhaler is likely to have *some* impact on 6-min walk distance in the population. The 95% confidence interval provides an estimate of *how much* impact is likely to be expected in the underlying population. The 95% confidence interval of 10 m – 70 m may be interpreted as, "we can be '95% confident' that the difference in 6-minute walk distance comparing the addition of the new inhaler to existing treatment could be as small as 10 meters or as large as 70 meters among *all* asthma patients who are similar to those in the trial."

In this example, the outcome variable, 6-min walk distance, is continuous (meaning it can take on a theoretically infinite number of values), promoting use of the *t*-test to compare mean values between the groups. The mean may be an appropriate summary measure if the characteristic of interest is continuous. However, if the outcome variable is categorical or binary, then a different test is needed.

15.1.2 Chi-Square Test

The chi-square test is a statistical test used to compare proportions between two (or more) different groups. Hypothesis testing using the chi-square test is conceptually similar to that of the *t*-test. For example, suppose a study observes a 5% incidence of middle ear infection among children who receive the pneumococcal vaccine and a 10% incidence of this infection among children who do not receive the vaccine. The chi-square test could be used to make an inference regarding potential differences in middle ear infection among all similar children in the population. The *p*-value from a chi-square test of these proportions would be interpreted as the probability of finding a 5% difference in middle ear infections, as observed in this study, or a more extreme difference, if there was no true difference in middle ear infection by pneumococcal vaccine status in the population. Taken together, the chi-square test and the *t*-test cover many situations in clinical research studies.

Table 15.2 Examples of statistical procedures for noncontinuous, nonbinary data

Type of data	Example characteristic	Statistical procedure
Counts	Number of heart failure exacerbations	Poisson regression
Censored survival data	Median survival	Kaplan-Meier estimation
Survival time	Overall survival	Logrank test
Odds ratio	Relative odds of multiple sclerosis	Logistic regression

Table 15.3 End-of-study systolic blood pressure results

Treatment	Number of people	Mean end-of-study systolic blood pressure (mmHg)	Standard deviation (mmHg)
Medication one	800	136	12
Medication two	800	139	11
Medication three	800	141	13
Medication four	800	134	11

ANOVA p-value <0.001

15.1.3 Hypothesis Tests for Other Types of Study Data

Other study characteristics may not be binary or continuous. Such data require different statistical procedures to obtain valid p-values and confidence intervals, shown in Table 15.2.

The interpretation of statistical testing for these types of data are analogous to those described for the t-test and chi-square test. Specifically, p-values obtained from these tests represent the probability of obtaining the sample (study) data given no true difference in the characteristic of interest in the underlying population.

15.1.4 Multiple Sample Hypothesis Tests

In some instances, statistical testing is needed to compare results among more than two groups. For example, investigators may wish to compare the impact of *four* different antihypertensive medications on end-of-study systolic blood pressure in a randomized trial, shown in Table 15.3.

The ANOVA test is used to compare mean values among more than two groups. The null hypothesis for the ANOVA test is that the mean values are equal among *all of the groups* in the underlying population. The interpretation of this ANOVA p-value is "if the four antihypertensive medications have equal effects on systolic blood pressure among all similar people, then the chance of observing these different end-of-study systolic blood pressures, or more extremely different systolic blood pressures, is <0.1%." The results of the ANOVA test imply that *at least one of these mean blood pressure values is different from the others in the population*, but do not inform as to which particular group may be different. The ANOVA test is often used as a "first pass" to check for significant differences among several groups.

15.2   An Imperfect System

Statistical hypothesis testing is not foolproof. A research study may falsely declare an association to be "statistically significant" when such an association does not actually exist in the underlying population. Such errors often occur due to chance and are exacerbated by performing multiple hypothesis tests on the same study data. Conversely, a study may observe and report a statistically nonsignificant result when in fact the association of interest is truly present in the population. Such errors can also arise from chance, but their likelihood is strongly influenced by the number of participants in the study (sample size), the strength of the association in the population (effect size), and the degree of variability in the outcome characteristic of interest.

15.2.1   Type I Error

For statistical hypothesis tests, the p-value returns the probability of observing a particular sample result, or a more extreme result, if a preconceived null hypothesis about the population is true. Given a "small" p-value (low probability of the null hypothesis), the null hypothesis is rejected and the alternative hypothesis is declared (most likely) to be true, implying that there is *some* effect or association in the population. But what defines a "small" p-value? A threshold value of 0.05 is typically used to define statistical significance in clinical research studies. That is, if the observed p-value is less than 0.05, then the null hypothesis is rejected and statistical significance declared.

Applying *any* p-value threshold implies that "statistical significance" will sometimes be observed even if the null hypothesis is true, due to chance. If the significance level is set to 0.05, then there is a 5% chance of observing a statistically significant result even if there is no true difference or association in the underlying population. For instance, if 100 randomized trials were conducted to compare the effect of two identical medications on depression scores, then five of these trials would be expected to observe a "statistically significant" difference between the two groups even though the medications are identical and must have the same effect on depression scores in the population.

A *type I error* occurs when a hypothesis test declares a study result to be statistically significant, yet the null hypothesis is true (no actual difference in the population). *Type I errors are an important motivation for replicating the results of research studies.* If there is a 5% chance of a type I error occurring in one study, then the chance of two independent studies finding a statistically significant result when no true population difference exists is only 0.5% * 0.5% = 0.25%.

Studies that perform multiple hypothesis tests on the same data are particularly prone to type I errors. Consider a study that explores many potential risk factors for liver cancer. Because each individual hypothesis test carries a type I error rate of 5% under the significance threshold of 0.05, every 20 hypothesis tests would be expected to yield one significant result due to chance alone, even if none of the evaluated risk factors are truly associated with cancer in the population. One approach to this *problem of multiple comparisons* is called the *Bonferroni correction*. This procedure limits the experiment-wide type I error rate to 5% by setting a more stringent *p*-value threshold for declaring a "significant" result. For example, if a study tests 12 potential risk factors for liver cancer, then the Bonferroni *p*-value threshold for declaring any individual risk factor to be significant would not be 0.05 but instead 0.05/12 = 0.0042.

The problem of multiple comparisons is of particular importance in studies of multifaceted individual-level data, such as genomics, proteomics, and metabolomics. These studies may evaluate thousands or millions of genetic variants, proteins, and small molecules to test for associations with disease. For example, genome-wide association studies often assess millions of genetic variants for associations with specific outcomes. Under a significance threshold of 0.05, 5% of these tests would be expected to be false positives, potentially yielding tens of thousands of false associations (association found to be significant in the study, but no true association actually exists in the population). Such studies strive to evaluate the largest possible number of people, replicate positive findngs in other studies, and control for type I error by setting an extremely low *p*-value threshold for declaring significance, such as 10^{-8} (*p*-value <0.00000001). However, setting a more stringent *p*-value threshold may engender the opposite problem: declaring an association to be nonsignificant when in fact the association truly exists in the underlying population (see type II error below). Specialized statistical procedures are often used in such studies to balance the likelihood of type I and type II errors.

15.2.2   Type II Error

A *type II error* occurs when a hypothesis test declares a study result to be statistically nonsignificant, yet a true difference or association exists in the population. Type II errors result in missing potentially important associations due to chance. For example, the study of liver cancer risk factors may observe that the consumption of more than two alcoholic beverages per day is associated with a 10% greater incidence of cancer: relative risk = 1.1; *p*-value = 0.15. Based on this *p*-value, the study would declare no significant association between consumption of more than two alcoholic beverages per day and cancer. Yet, based on findings reported from other studies, this risk factor *is* likely to be associated with liver cancer in the underlying population from which the study participants were selected.

15.3   Power

Research studies strive to collect enough data to detect important associations or effects. Power represents the ability a study to detect some pre-specified difference or association in the underlying population. Specifically, power is defined as the probability that a particular study will *not* make a type II error, given an assumption about the size of the difference or association in the population. Type II errors often occur due to *inadequate study power*.

Study power is frequently calculated before conducting a study to determine the number of participants who would need to be recruited.

Example 15.2 Researchers design a randomized trial to compare the effect of two novel antihypertensive medications on blood pressure. Before conducting the trial, the researchers decide that a 10-mmHg difference in systolic blood pressure between the treatment groups is "clinically important." They conduct power calculations to determine that a study of 192 people will have 80% power and a study of 258 people will have 90% power to detect this prespecified 10 mmHg difference in systolic blood pressure.

The 80% power in this example can be interpreted as, "even if there is a true 10 mmHg difference in systolic blood pressure between the two study medications in the population, there is still a 20% chance that a study of 192 people will return a statistically nonsignificant result (type II error)." A study of 258 people is only 10% likely to make a type II error in this setting.

What factors might cause a study to miss true associations in the population? Study power is affected by four major characteristics: sample size (N), the magnitude of effect in the population (often the difference in mean values between groups), the variability of the outcome measurements (σ), and the significance level of the test (α; usually fixed at 0.05). These factors influence the interpretation of p-values obtained for a given study result, warranting discussion of each factor more carefully.

15.3.1 Sample Size (N)

Statistical power increases with increasing sample size, such that a study of 5000 people is considerably more likely to detect a statistically significant result compared to a study of 500 people if the result is truly present in the population. An implication of this relationship is that *large studies have the ability to detect very small effects that may be statistically significant but clinically irrelevant*. For this reason, the importance of study results should be appraised by not only the p-value but also by the magnitude of the effect and the corresponding confidence interval.

Consider a hypothetical large randomized trial that detects a statistically significant 0.03-mmHg difference in end-of-study systolic blood pressure between two medications (p-value = 0.01; 95% confidence interval +0.01, +0.05 mmHg). Such a small difference in systolic blood pressure is clinically inconsequential. Additionally, the upper limit of the 95% confidence interval (+0.05 mmHg) suggests that a clinically important difference in the underlying population is unlikely.

On the other hand, a smaller study may find that a new antihypertension medication lowers systolic blood pressure by 15 mmHg compared with conventional medications (p-value = 0.15; 95% confidence interval −2, +32 mmHg). The confidence interval does not exclude the possibility that the new medication has no impact on systolic blood pressure in the underlying population but also does not exclude the possibility of clinically important (large) effects. The study may have been under-powered; additional studies that recruit more participants would be needed to better estimate the true impact of the new medication in the underlying population.

It should also be noted that large study populations are more likely to contain people who have unusual characteristics in the underlying population. For example, if a medication causes a rare adverse effect in 0.2% of the population, then a study of 100 participants is unlikely to contain such a person, but a study of 5000 people will, on average, contain ten such people. The study of rare side effects is a strength of observational studies of medication use (pharmacoepidemiology studies), which have the opportunity to evaluate very large numbers of treated patients.

15.3.2   Effect Size (μ)

Statistical power increases fairly dramatically when the true magnitude of effect in the population is large. For example, a small study may be adequately powered to demon-strate a statistically significant effect for a breakthrough cancer drug that prolongs disease-free survival by 50%. In contrast, very large numbers of study participants are needed to adequately power studies to detect subtle treatment effects, for example, studies comparing the effect of two medications within the same class. Tables 15.4 and 15.5 present sample size calculations for three hypothetical risk factors for hyper-tension that are strongly, moderately, and weakly associated with this outcome.

Table 15.4 Sample size needed to detect associations with hypertension

Risk factor	Incidence of hypertension (%)		Relative risk	Number of people needed to detect significant association[a]
	Risk factor present	Risk factor absent		
One	40	20	40/20 = 2.0	164
Two	30	20	30/20 = 1.5	588
Three	24	20	24/20 = 1.2	3366

[a]Assumes 80% study power and a p-value threshold of 0.05 to declare significance (alpha)

Table 15.5 Sample size needed to detect associations with systolic blood pressure

Risk factor	Mean systolic blood pressure ± standard deviation (mmHg)		Difference in mean systolic blood pressure (mmHg)	Number of people needed to detect significant association[a]
	Risk factor present	Risk factor absent		
One	140 ± 20	130 ± 20	10	128
Two	135 ± 20	130 ± 20	5	506
Three	132 ± 20	130 ± 20	2	3142

[a]Assumes 80% study power and a p-value threshold of 0.05 to declare significance (alpha)

A statistically significant association between relatively strong risk factor one and hypertension could be detected in a study of only 164 people (82 in each group). On the other hand, a study of 3366 people would be needed to detect a statistically significant association between relatively weak risk factor three and hypertension. A similarly large number of subjects would be required to detect smaller differences in mean systolic blood pressure associated with risk factor three. Given a fixed number of subjects, studies of relatively strong risk factors will have considerably greater power to detect statistically significant associations than studies of weaker risk factors.

The relationship of effect size with study power highlights the challenge of evaluating all-cause mortality as an outcome in randomized trials. The inclusion of mortality as a study outcome may substantially dilute the effects of interventions that target a single disease pathway. For example, several randomized trials have compared different treatment strategies among patients with critical illness, including alternative approaches to volume resuscitation, varying combinations of vasopressor agents, the administration of systemic steroids, and scheduled red blood cell transfusions. None of these trials have observed statistically significant differences in all-cause mortality comparing one treatment strategy to another. However, all-cause mortality in critical illness is influenced by a wide-range of conditions and biological pathways, many of which are unlikely to be related to any single intervention. The impact of any one of these individual treatment strategies on all-cause mortality is likely to be very small, requiring extremely large sample sizes to detect significant associations.

15.3.3   Variability (σ)

Statistical power increases with decreasing variability of the outcome characteristic. In other words, a more tightly spaced distribution of the outcome variable will yield greater statistical power compared with a more widely spaced distribution. Consider two hypothetical randomized trials that each detect a 7 mmHg difference in systolic blood pressure between two antihypertensive medications, shown in Fig. 15.1.

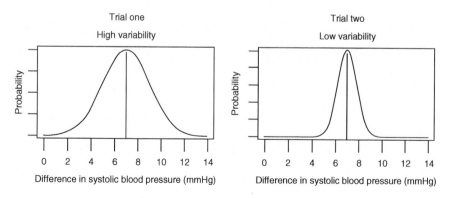

Fig. 15.1 Difference in systolic blood pressure for two hypothetical clinical trials

In the first trial, the distribution of the difference in systolic blood pressures is relatively spread out, suggesting a heterogeneous response to the medications across the study population. In contrast, the difference in systolic blood pressures between the two medications is more tightly spaced in the second trial, suggesting more consistent effects. The second trial has greater power to demonstrate that the observed 7-mmHg difference in mean systolic blood pressure is statistically significant.

In general, studies that evaluate highly variable outcomes will have less power to demonstrate statistical significance compared with studies that assess more consistent outcome measures.

15.3.4 Significance Level (α)

The significance level is the p-value threshold used to define a statistically significant test. This value is usually fixed at 0.05 for clinical research studies. However, it is useful to note that study power will increase if the significance level is set to a value greater than 0.05, as is sometimes done in exploratory studies or phase II clinical trials, which may be underpowered due to relatively small numbers of participants. Conversely, power will decrease if the significance level is set to a value less than 0.05, for example, when correcting for multiple comparisons. This property makes sense in that it will be easier to detect a "statistically significant" result when the threshold to declare significance is set to a higher value.

Chapter 16
Linear Regression

Summary of Learning Points

16.1 Regression is used to estimate the association between two or more study variables.

16.2 Univariate linear regression

16.2.1 The univariate linear regression equation is described by: $Y = \beta_0 + \beta_1 \times (X)$

16.2.2 A *residual* in a linear regression model is the difference between the observed study data and the predicted value from the model.

16.2.3 A *coefficient* in a linear regression model describes the mean difference in the outcome variable associated with a one-unit difference in the predictor variable.

16.3 Diagnostic tests assess whether the fitted regression model accurately fits the study data.

16.3.1 Nonlinear study data may not be well described by any linear regression model.

16.3.2 An outlier is a data point that is located far away from most of the other data points.

16.3.3 An influential data point has a large impact on the slope of the regression line.

16.3.4 Extrapolating the regression equation beyond the observed data can lead to error.

16.4 Multiple linear regression

16.4.1 The multiple linear regression equation is described by: $Y = \beta_0 + \beta_1 \times (X_1) + \beta_2 \times (X_2) \ldots$

16.4.2 Each coefficient in a multiple linear regression model describes the mean difference in the outcome variable associated with a one-unit difference in the predictor variable, holding the other variables in the model constant.

16.4.3 The null hypothesis for a coefficient in a linear regression model is that the coefficient = 0.

© Springer Nature Switzerland AG 2019
B. Kestenbaum, *Epidemiology and Biostatistics*,
https://doi.org/10.1007/978-3-319-96644-1_16

16.5 Regression models can be used to assess confounding and effect modification.

    16.5.1 The presence of confounding is suspected when the coefficient of interest changes meaningfully after adding a characteristic to the regression model.

    16.5.2 The presence of effect modification is suspected when the coefficient of interest differs by a modifying variable in a regression model that includes a product term.

Regression is a mathematical procedure used to estimate the association between two or more study variables. *Multiple regression* is a widely used tool in clinical research studies to adjust for many confounding characteristics simultaneously.

16.1   Describing the Association Between Two Variables

Example 16.1 Vitamin D may reduce chronic inflammation by modulating the transcription of specific genes related to lymphocyte functions. A hypothetical cross-sectional study examines the association of circulating vitamin D levels with interleukin 6 (IL-6), a pro-inflammatory cytokine. Researchers collect blood samples from 50 healthy volunteers and measure serum concentrations of IL-6 and 25-hydroxyvitamin D, the circulating storage form of vitamin D.

    Data for the 50 study participants is shown in Fig. 16.1.

    Visual inspection of this plot suggests that higher serum 25-hydroxyvitamin D levels tend to track with lower IL-6 levels, consistent with the study hypothesis. However, the scatter plot provides only descriptive evidence. There is no formal *test* of the association between serum 25-hydroxyvitamin D and IL-6 levels. Moreover, the scatter plot does not quantify the *size* of this association. In other words, about how much lower are serum IL-6 levels per unit higher 25-hydroxyvitamin D levels?

    Recall that the *t*-test is used to compare mean values between two different groups. The *t*-test could be applied here by dividing the continuous vitamin D levels into two groups. For example, some experts recommend defining vitamin D deficiency by a serum 25-hydroxyvitamin D level <15 ng/ml. Based on this definition, the *t*-test can be applied to the association of vitamin D deficiency with serum IL-6 levels.

Vitamin D status	Number of people	Mean IL-6 level	Standard deviation
Deficient (<15 ng/ml)	18	2.4 pg/ml	1.6 pg/ml
Replete (≥15 ng/ml)	32	1.7 pg/ml	1.1 pg/ml
		T-test *p*-value = 0.11	

    The interpretation of this *p*-value is, "if mean serum IL-6 levels are equal among vitamin D deficient and vitamin D replete people in the underlying population, then the chance of observing these different mean IL-6 values, or even more extremely

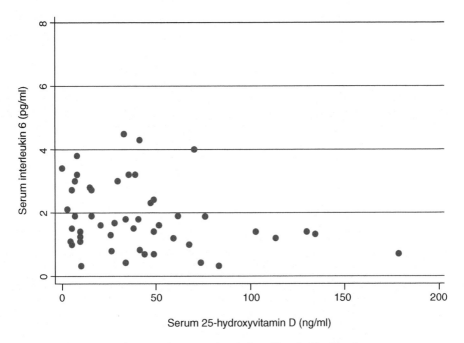

Fig. 16.1 Scatter plot of serum 25-hydroxyvitamin D and interleukin-6 levels

different values, by vitamin D status is 11%." This *p*-value is insufficiently small to reject the null hypothesis.

The use of a *t*-test in this situation involves compromise. The vitamin D data must be divided into two separate groups based on a specifc cut point. Other definitions of vitamin D deficiency have been proposed, such as a 25-hydroxyvitamin D level <20 ng/ml. The results of the *t*-test will differ depending on the cut point selected to define vitamin D deficiency. Moreover, dividing the data into only two groups restricts analysis of the full measured range of serum 25-hydroxyvitamin D values. A better method to describe these study data is linear regression, which can quantify the continuous association of interest and test for statistical significance.

16.2   Univariate Linear Regression

16.2.1   The Linear Regression Equation

All lines are characterized by having some *slope* and some *intercept* (defined as the *y*-value when $X = 0$), described by the general equation:

$$Y = mX + b;$$

where *m* is the slope and *b* is the intercept.

A regression line relating serum 25-hydroxyvitamin D and IL-6 levels would assume the form:

$$\text{IL-6 level} = m \times (25\text{-hydroxyvitamin D level}) + b$$

Standard parlance for regression analyses is to use the terms "β_1" to represent the slope and "β_0" to represent the intercept. So, the regression equation can be rewritten as:

$$\text{IL-6} = \beta_0 + \beta_1 \times (25\text{-hydroxyvitamin D});$$

where β_0 is the intercept and β_1 is the slope.

The beta terms in the equation are also called *coefficients*.

Each possible set of slope (β_1) and intercept (β_0) values describes a unique line relating serum 25-hydroxyvitamin D with serum IL-6 levels. One of these lines will most closely fit the observed study data. In other words, there exists a best possible pair of β_0 and β_1 values for which the resulting regression line lies closest to all of the data points in the study. The mathematical methods (calculus) used to find the best fitting intercept and slope are beyond the scope of this book. Statistical software packages will quickly find the solution for a regression line from a set of raw data.

Entering the 25-hydroxyvitamin D and IL-6 study data into a computer program yields the best fitting intercept and slope coefficients of 2.4 and −0.01, respectively.

$$\text{IL-6 level} = 2.4 + (-0.01) \times (25\text{-hydroxyvitamin D level})$$

The resolved regression equation, which is also called the *model*, is presented in Fig. 16.2.

16.2.2 Residuals and the Sum of Squares

The fitted regression equation can be used to *predict* the average serum IL-6 level based on a given 25-hydroxyvitamin D level. For example, a study participant has a measured serum 25-hydroyvitamin D level of 35 ng/ml. Based on the linear regression equation, this participant's predicted IL-6 level would be:

$$\text{IL-6 level} = 2.4 + (-0.01) \times (25\text{-hydroxyvitamin D level})$$
$$= 2.4 - (0.01) \times (35) = 2.1 \, \text{pg/ml}$$

A *residual* is defined as the difference between the actual study data and the value predicted from a fitted regression equation. For the participant with a serum 25-hydroyvitamin D level of 35 ng/ml, their actual measured IL-6 level is 3.0 pg/ml. The residual for this person would be:

$$\text{Residual} = \text{observed value} - \text{predicted value} = 3.0 \, \text{pg/ml} - 2.1 \, \text{pg/ml} = 0.9 \, \text{pg/ml}$$

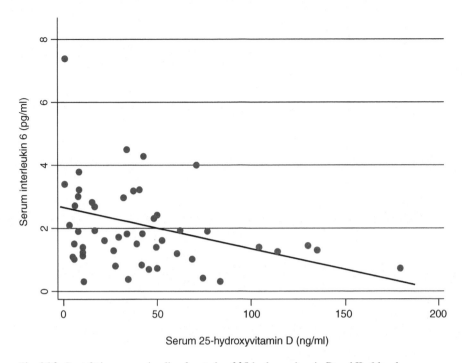

Fig. 16.2 Best fitting regression line for study of 25-hydroxyvitamin D and IL-6 levels

Residuals can be viewed graphically as the vertical distance between the measured study data and the regression line, shown in Fig. 16.3.

The participant of interest is represented by the arrow in the figure. This person's residual is represented by the vertical distance between their actual measured IL-6 level and their predicted IL-6 level on the regression line.

In aggregate, the residuals describe how closely a regression line fits the observed study data. Specifically, the sum of all of the residuals describes how closely a fitted regression line lies to all the data points. In practice, each residual is typically squared before summation. Consequently, the best fitting regression line is defined as the line that has the *lowest sum of squared residuals*. In other words, the best fitting regression line lies closest to all the data points, where "close" is measured in squared distance.

16.2.3 Interpreting Continuous Covariates from a Linear Regression Model

The fitted regression equation can be used to quantify the association between serum 25-hydroxyvitamin and IL-6 levels:

$$\text{IL-6 level} = 2.4 + (-0.01) \times (\text{25-hydroxyvitamin D level})$$

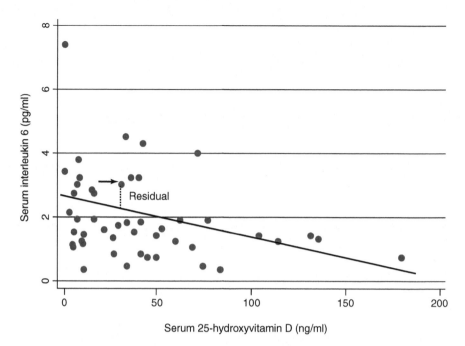

Fig. 16.3 Residual for a data point in a linear regression model

$$\left(\begin{array}{c}\text{IL-6 levels are measured in pg / ml and 25-hydroxyvitamin}\\\text{D levels are measured in ng / ml}\end{array}\right)$$

The coefficient of −0.01 can be interpreted as, "each 1 ng/ml higher serum 25-hydroxyvitamin D level is associated with, on average, a 0.01 pg/ml lower IL-6 level." The sign (positive or negative) before the coefficient specifies whether an association is positive (higher values of the predictor variable associated with higher values of the outcome) or negative (higher values of the predictor variable associated with lower values of the outcome). In this instance, the coefficient for 25-hydroxyvitamin D is negative indicating an inverse association.

The fitted linear regression equation can also be used to predict the expected difference in serum IL-6 levels between two people who have differing serum levels of 25-hydroxyvitamin D. Consider two study participants who have serum 25-hydroxyvitamin D levels of 20 ng/ml and 10 ng/ml. Based on the best fitting regression equation:

$$\text{Person one : Predicted mean IL-6 level} = 2.4 - (0.01) \times (20) = 2.2 \text{ pg / ml}$$

$$\text{Person two : Predicted mean IL-6 level} = 2.4 - (0.01) \times (10) = 2.3 \text{ pg / ml}$$

Person one has a predicted serum IL-6 level that is, on average, 0.1 pg/ml lower than that of person two. This predicted 0.1 pg/ml difference applies to *any* 10 ng/ml difference in serum 25-hydroyvitamin levels in the study, because the regression model assumes a constant linear association between these characteristics. Consequently, a person with a serum 25-hydroyvitamin level of 60 ng/ml would be expected to have an IL-6 level that is, on average, 0.1 pg/ml lower that of a person with a level of 50 ng/ml.

16.2.4   Interpreting Binary Covariates from Linear Regression Equations

To use binary variables in regression equations, one category of the variable is assigned the value of 1, and the other category is assigned the value of 0. For example, a linear regression equation to relate sex with serum IL-6 levels can be constructed by assigning men a value of 1 and women a value of 0, shown in Fig. 16.4.

The best fitting regression equation for these study data is:

$$\text{IL-6 level} = 1.5 + 0.67 \times (\text{sex});$$

where sex = 1 for men and 0 for women.

How can we interpret the results from this model? For each 1-unit increase in the variable representing sex, serum IL-6 levels are, on average, 0.67 pg/ml higher.

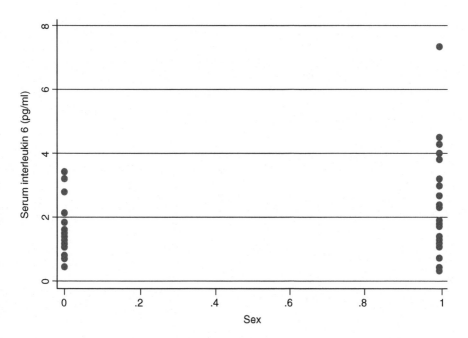

Fig. 16.4 Association of sex with interleukin-6 levels

The sex variable is defined such that a one-unit increase is the same as comparing men to women. So, the results of the regression model indicate that IL-6 levels are, on average, 0.67 pg/ml higher among men compared to women. We can examine the study data to check whether this finding is in fact true.

	Mean IL-6 level (pg/ml)
Men	2.17
Women	1.50
Difference in means	0.67

The regression equation exactly predicts the mean difference in IL-6 levels by sex. Note that because there were only two categories, this analysis could also be performed using a *t*-test. The test of whether the slope is significant (whether 0.67 is statistically different from 0) is identical to the *t*-test for a difference in mean IL-6 levels between men and women.

16.3   Diagnostics

The previous interpretations of results obtained from regression models assumed that the model reasonably described the observed study data. The sum of squares procedure will identify the best fitting line to the observed data among all possible lines. However, the fitted regression line is an artificial construct that does not go through most (if any) of the actual data points. There is no assurance that the best fitting line will accurately describe the study data *in any absolute sense*. In practice, statistical procedures are used to confirm the overall fit of a regression equation by subjective inspection of the study data, hypothesis testing, and consideration of potentially influential data points.

16.3.1   *Absolute Versus Relative Fit*

A simple first procedure is to compare the fitted regression line to a horizontal line drawn through the mean of the study data. For example, the mean IL-6 level in the vitamin D study is 2.0 pg/ml. Figure 16.5 depicts comparison of the fitted regression line (study hypothesis) to a horizontal line through the mean of the data (null hypothesis).

The sum of squared residuals is used to measure how closely each of these lines lies to all of the data points. These sums are then compared using the concept of hypothesis testing introduced earlier. In this example, the null hypothesis would be, "there is no linear association between serum 25-hydroxyvitamin D and IL-6 levels in the underlying population." This is equivalent to the statement that the best fitting

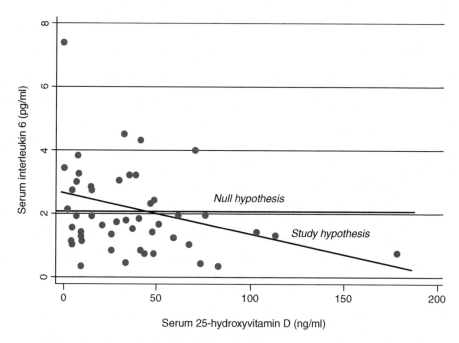

Fig. 16.5 Comparison of regression line to horizontal line through the mean

line has a slope equal to 0. The study (alternative) hypothesis is that there is *some* linear association between serum 25-hydroxyvitamin D and IL-6 levels in the population, or that the best fitting line has a slope that is not equal to zero. If the fitted regression line is found to have a significantly smaller sum of squared residuals than the horizontal line, then the regression line more accurately explains the observed study data and the null hypothesis of no association is rejected.

16.3.2 Nonlinear Associations

The linear regression model represents the best possible *line* that can be fit to the observed study data. However, there is no guarantee that study data are well described by *any* line. The fit of a linear regression equation can be assessed by comparing the equation with a more complex function, shown in Fig. 16.6.

   The sum of squared residuals is used to determine how closely each equation fits the observed study data. In this example, the sum of squared residuals for the best fitting line and best fitting complex function are statistically similar, implying that the linear equation fits the observed serum 25-hydroxyvitamin D and IL-6 data reasonably well.

Example 16.2 Control of blood pressure is an important for managing acute stroke. Inappropriately low blood pressures can extend infract size by exacerbating ischemia, and inappropriately high blood pressures can increase the risk of intracerebral

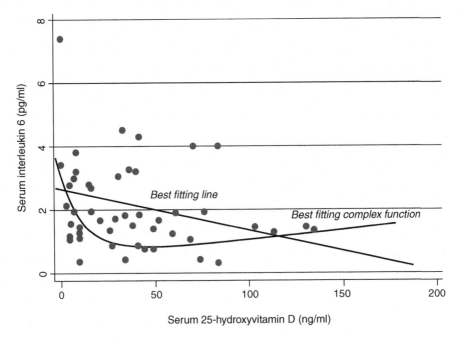

Fig. 16.6 Test of linear association between 25-hydroxyvitamin D and interleukin-6 levels

bleeding. Researchers use a linear regression model to examine the association between systolic blood pressure and cerebral infarct size in a hypothetical study of 90 patients with acute stroke. They report that each 10-mmHg higher systolic blood pressure is associated with a 0.4-mm^3 smaller cerebral infarct size. Based on this finding, the researchers conclude that, "systolic blood pressure should be maintained as high as possible in acute stroke to avoid extension of infarct size."

The use of linear regression implies that a best fitting linear model was used to obtain these study results. However, there is no assurance that a line accurately describes the study data in any absolute sense. The blood pressure and infarct size data are presented graphically in Fig. 16.7.

Visual inspection of these data reveals that the association between systolic blood pressure and infarct size is *not* well explained by *any* line. Cerebral infarct size appears to be smallest for systolic blood pressures between 130 and 140 mmHg, with larger infarcts observed for both higher and lower blood pressures. Although a best fitting line can always be forced through the study data, it is important to consider whether a linear association appropriately describes the association of interest. In this example, a U-shaped equation better describes the systolic blood pressure and infarct size data, shown in Fig. 16.8.

The conclusion that systolic blood pressure should be maintained at higher levels in acute stroke to minimize infarct size is faulty, based on the interpretation of a regression line that poorly fits the observed study data.

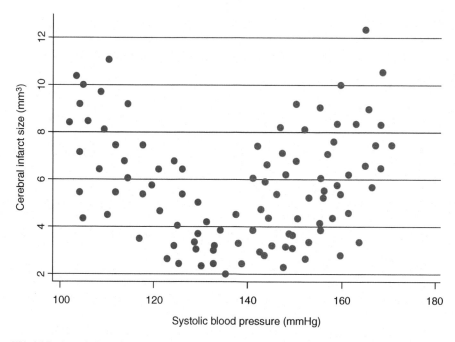

Fig. 16.7 Association of systolic blood pressure with cerebral infarct size in acute stroke

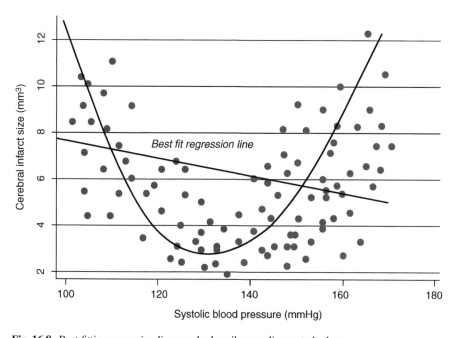

Fig. 16.8 Best fitting regression line poorly describes nonlinear study data

16.3.3   Influential Points

The best fitting regression line is defined by the smallest sum of the squared distances between the observed data points and the line. This process implies that not all of the data points will contribute equally in terms of their influence on the slope of the fitted regression line. Consider the addition of three new data points to the original study of serum 25-hydroxyvitamin D and IL-6 levels, shown in Fig. 16.9.

Data points #1 and #2 have the greatest potential to influence the fitted line, because their x-value lies far away from most of the other data points (these people have extremely high serum 25-hydroxyvitamin D levels). Data point #1 also has an atypically high serum IL-6 level. The combination of an extreme x- *and* an extreme y-value for data point #1 will result in a meaningful change in the slope of the fitted regression line. The dashed line in the figure represents the best fitting regression line with inclusion of data point #1, and the solid line represents the best fitting line excluding this data point. In this instance, a single observation causes a marked decrease in the size of the association between 25-hydroxyvitamin D and IL-6 levels (slope). A data point that meaningfully influences the slope of the regression line is called an *influential point*.

On the other hand, data point #2 has only a small influence on the fitted regression line, because the y-value for this point is similar to those of the surrounding values. Analogously, data point #3 is unlikely to be influential, because the x-value for this point lies close to the other x-values in the dataset. Data points #2 and #3 would simply be called *outliers*, because they reside far away from the other data points but have little impact on the fitted regression line.

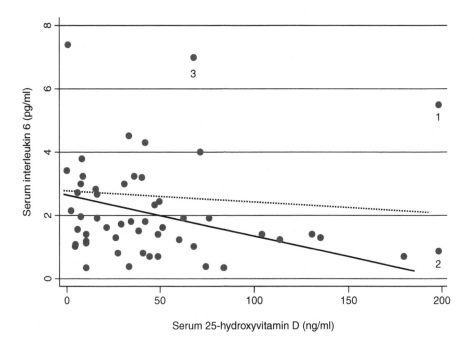

Fig. 16.9   Influence of extreme data points on the fitted regression line

Single data points with high influence are concerning, because effect sizes and statistical inference can be driven by only a small number of such points, or even a single point. A first step for addressing extreme data points is to certify that these values are valid. For example, extreme IL-6 or 25-hydroxyvitamin D values could be caused by errors in the laboratory assay or miscoding of the study samples. It is also possible that the extremely high serum 25-hydroxyvitamin D levels were caused by high-dose vitamin D supplementation. For extreme data points that are certified to be valid, the degree of influence can be calculated by comparing the fitted regression equations with and without removal of the outlying data point. The results of such tests should be reported in the study. The decision to remove highly influential data points from the analyses is subjective. In this instance, removing data point #1 will provide a more accurate description of the association between serum 25-hydroxyvitamin D and IL-6 levels for people who have "typical" vitamin D levels. More data are needed to accurately assess this association among people who have extremely high values of 25-hydroxyvitamin D.

16.3.4   Extrapolating the Regression Equation Beyond the Observed Data

The observed study data are used to determine the best fitting linear regression equation. However, there is no guarantee that a given equation will provide valid prediction for data outside the range of observed values. Extrapolating prediction from regression equations beyond the observed data can lead to erroneous findings. A tragic example is estimation of the amount of damage to the rubber O-rings used to seal booster rocket joints in the space shuttle Challenger (Fig. 16.10).

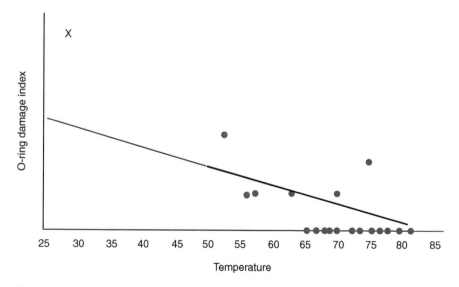

Fig. 16.10 Association between temperature and O-ring damage

The circles represent data from previous shuttle launches under relatively temperate conditions. The dark line represents the fitted linear regression model to the previously observed data. Extrapolation of the regression line to predict O-ring damage for much colder temperatures (dashed line) is invalid, because no previous launches were performed at such temperatures. The Challenger launch at 29 degrees Fahrenheit resulted in far greater O-ring damage than anticipated (represented by the X in the figure).

16.4   Multiple Linear Regression

16.4.1   Definition of the Multiple Regression Model

Suppose that we are interested in evaluating how *two* different characteristics are associated with serum IL-6 levels? The regression equation for one predictor variable was defined as:

$$Y = \beta_0 + \beta_1 \times (\text{predictor})$$

The regression equation can be extended for multiple predictor variables:

$$Y = \beta_0 + \beta_1 \times (\text{predictor 1}) + \beta_2 \times (\text{predictor 2}) + \beta_3 \times (\text{predictor 3})\ldots$$

For example, let's say we are interested in the association of serum 25-hydroxyvitamin D levels *and* sex with serum IL-6 levels. The following equation can be constructed for this purpose:

$$\text{IL-6} = \beta_0 + \beta_1 \times (\text{vitamin D}) + \beta_2 \times (\text{sex});$$

where sex is arbitrarily defined as 1 for men and 0 for women.

The resulting equation no longer represents a line, but rather a three-dimensional surface, because each serum IL-6 level predicted by the equation is associated with a specific vitamin D level and a specific sex (male or female). Multiple regression is typically performed using a computer. The dataset containing the observed study values of IL-6, 25-hydroxyvitamin D, and sex for each participant is entered into a computer, which determines the best fitting regression equation. In other words, the computer finds optimal values for the coefficients β_0, β_1, and β_2, such that the sum of squared residuals is as small as possible.

The best fitting linear equation to these study data is described by:

$$\text{IL-6} = 1.97 - 0.01 \times (\text{25-hydroxyvitamin D}) + 0.70 \times (\text{sex})$$

The residuals from a multiple regression model are calculated in the same way as for a univariate regression model. A predicted IL-6 value can be calculated from the model for each study participant based on his or her 25-hydroxyvitamin D level and sex. For example, a female participant who has a serum 25-hydroxyvitamin D level of 10 ng/ml would have the following predicted IL-6 value:

$$\text{IL-6} = 1.97 - 0.01 \times (25\text{-hydroxyvitamin D}) + 0.70 \times (\text{sex})$$
$$= 1.97 - 0.01 \times (10) + 0.7 \times (0) = 1.87$$

The residual for this person is defined as the difference between their actual measured IL-6 level and their model-predicted IL-6 value of 1.87 pg/ml.

The procedures used to fit and assess multiple linear regression models are analogous to those described for the univariate model:

1. Use the sum of squares procedure to find the best fitting linear equation to the study data.
2. Appraise how well the derived equation fits the study data in an absolute sense.
3. Check for possible influential values.

For the purposes of this example, we will assume that the fitted model represents a reasonably good fit to the study data and will proceed with interpretation.

16.4.2   Interpreting Results from the Multiple Regression Model

16.4.2.1   Obtaining Estimated Values for a Particular Set of Data

The fitted multiple regression model can be used to predict the value of the outcome variable for any combination of predictor variables. For a hypothetical *male* participant who has a 25-hydroxyvitamin D level of 10 ng/ml:

$$\text{Mean IL-6} = 1.97 - 0.01 \times (\text{vitamin D}) + 0.70 \times (\text{sex})$$
$$= 1.97 - 0.01 \times (10) + 0.70 \times (1) = 2.57 \, \text{pg} / \text{ml}$$

For a hypothetical *female* participant who had a 25-hydroxyvitamin D level of 30 ng/ml:

$$\text{Mean IL-6} = 1.97 - 0.01 \times (\text{vitamin D}) + 0.70 \times (\text{sex})$$
$$= 1.97 - 0.01 \times (30) + 0.70 \times (0) = 1.67 \, \text{pg} / \text{ml}$$

16.4.2.2   Obtaining Relative Differences in the Outcome Variable by a Covariate

A more common question regarding the study data might be, "what is the difference in serum IL-6 levels comparing men to women, independent of their vitamin D status?" In other words, "what is the association between sex and IL-6 levels, holding vitamin D levels constant?"

According to the model, the average IL-6 level for *any* man in the study is:

$$\text{Mean IL-6} = 1.97 - 0.01 \times (\text{vitamin D}) + 0.70 \times (1)$$

According to the model, the average IL-6 level for *any* woman in the study is:

$$\text{Mean IL-6} = 1.97 - 0.01 \times (\text{vitamin D}) + 0.70 \times (0)$$

Consequently, the *difference* in IL-6 levels, comparing men to women, is:

$$1.97 - 0.01 \times (\text{vitamin D}) + 0.70 \times (1) - 1.97 - 0.01 \times (\text{vitamin D}) + 0.70 \times (0)$$
$$= 0.70 \text{pg} / \text{ml}$$

All of the terms will cancel out, leaving a difference of 0.70 pg/ml.

This result can be interpreted as, "men have serum IL-6 levels that are, on average, 0.70 pg/ml higher than those of women, holding serum vitamin D levels constant."

Returning the original regression equation:

$$\text{IL-6} = 1.97 - 0.01 \times (\text{vitamin D}) + 0.70 \times (\text{sex})$$

As illustrated by the above example, the *individual coefficients from a multiple regression model represent the independent association between a predictor variable and the outcome variable, holding all other variables in the model constant.* This rule is used to interpret results of regression equations that have many predictor variables and demonstrates the use of multiple regression as a method to control for confounding.

Consider a more complex multiple regression equation that models serum IL-6 levels as a function of 25-hydroxyvitamin D levels, sex, age, smoking status, and LDL cholesterol levels. Again, the sex variable will be coded as 0 for women, 1 for men, and the smoking variable will be coded as 0 for a non-smoker, and 1 for a smoker. The general equation for this model is:

$$\text{Mean IL-6} = \beta_0 + \beta_1 \times (\text{vitamin D}) + \beta_2 \times (\text{sex}) + \beta_3 \times (\text{age})$$
$$+ \beta_4 \times (\text{smoke}) + \beta_5 \times (\text{LDL})$$

Using a computer to obtain the minimum sum of squared residuals returns a set of beta coefficients ($\beta_0 - \beta_5$) that most closely fits the study data:

$$\text{Mean IL-6} = 1.1 - 0.01 \times (\text{vitamin D}) + 0.7 \times (\text{sex}) + 0.02 \times (\text{age})$$
$$+ 0.4 \times (\text{smoke}) - 0.01 \times (\text{LDL})$$

The independent association between each predictor variable and the mean IL-6 level is specified by their specific coefficients in the model. For example,

- Each 1-year-older age is associated with an average 0.02 pg/ml higher serum IL-6 level, holding 25-hydroxyvitamin D levels, sex, smoking, and LDL cholesterol levels constant.
- For each 1 mg/dl greater LDL cholesterol levels, serum IL-6 levels are, on average, 0.01 pg/ml lower, holding 25-hydroxyvitamin D levels, sex, age, and smoking constant.
- Smokers have, on average, 0.4 pg/ml higher serum IL-6 levels compared to non-smokers, holding all of the other variables in the model constant.

The multiple regression equation has simultaneously adjusted for all of the specified characteristics in the model using all of the observed study data.

16.4.2.3 Interpreting Multiple Regression Results in Research Articles

Research articles do not typically report the specific multiple regression models used to obtain the study results. Instead, studies typically present the coefficients from these models in tabular form. For example, Table 16.1 presents results from a cross-sectional study that examined several potential risk factors in association with kidney function, measured by the glomerular filtration rate (GFR).
What model was used to obtain these study results?

- GFR $= \beta_0 + \beta_1 \times (\text{age}) + \beta_2 \times (\text{non - steroidal use}) + \beta_3 \times (\text{diabetes}) + \beta_4 \times (\text{hypertension})$

What coefficients were obtained for the fitted model?

- GFR $= 130 - 1.2 \times (\text{age}) - 6.0 \times (\text{non - steroidal use}) - 18.4 \times (\text{diabetes}) - 13.9 \times (\text{hypertension})$

where nonsteroidal use, diabetes, and hypertension are coded as 1 if these conditions are present and 0 if absent.
Note that there is no way to determine that the intercept is 130 from the data shown in Table 16.1.
What is the interpretation of the coefficient for diabetes (β_3) in this example?

- Given two people who are the same age, have the same use of non-steroidal medications (yes or no), and have the same hypertension status (yes or no), the presence of diabetes is associated with an estimated 18.4 ml/min lower GFR compared to the absence of diabetes. Stated another way, "diabetes is associated

Table 16.1 Adjusted associations of potential risk factors with kidney function

	Kidney function (GFR in ml/min)	95% confidence interval	P-value
Age (per year higher)	−1.2	(−0.8, −1.6)	<0.01
Nonsteroidal use	−6.0	(+2.0, −14.0)	0.11
Diabetes	−18.4	(−6.7, −30.1)	0.01
Hypertension	−13.9	(−3.5, −24.3)	0.02

Results are adjusted for all of the characteristics in the table with an estimated 18.4 ml/min lower GFR *after adjustment* for age, non-steroidal use, and hypertension."

What is the interpretation of the coefficient for age (β_1) in this example?

- The coefficient for age, a continuous characteristic, would be interpreted as, "each one-year older age is associated with an average 1.2 ml/min lower GFR holding non-steroidal use, diabetes, and hypertension status constant." The linear modeling of age implies that each ten-year difference in age is associated with a 12 ml/min lower GFR.

16.4.2.4   *P*-Values and Confidence Intervals for Regression Coefficients

For linear regression coefficients, the null hypothesis is that the coefficient is equal to 0, implying no association between the predictor variable and the outcome variable in the underlying population. The *p*-value of 0.01 for the diabetes coefficient in Table 16.1 can be interpreted as, "if there was no adjusted association between diabetes and GFR in the underlying population, then the chance of observing this adjusted −18.4 ml/min difference in GFR, or an even greater adjusted difference, is 1%." The results of this inference test imply that diabetes *is* likely to be associated with some adjusted difference in kidney function in the population.

The 95% confidence interval for the diabetes coefficient can be interpreted as, "if this experiment were repeated an infinite number of times, and a 95% confidence interval placed around each regression coefficient for diabetes, then 95% of the confidence intervals would contain the true adjusted association of diabetes with GFR in the population." We don't know whether this particular 95% confidence interval of (−6.7, −30.1) happens to be one of the confidence intervals that contains the true population value, but since 95% of such intervals contain this value, we can be "95% confident" that diabetes is associated with as little as a 6.7 ml/min lower GFR or as much as a 30.1 ml/min lower GFR in the underlying population after adjustment for age, nonsteroidal use, and hypertension.

16.5   Confounding and Effect Modification in Multiple Regression Models

Although the scientific concepts of confounding and effect modification were previously covered in Chaps. 10 and 11, we pause here to note how they can be viewed within a regression framework.

16.5.1   Confounding

Suppose we were interested in describing the association between height and serum IL-6 levels. We obtain the following best fitting linear regression equation to the study data:

$$\text{Mean IL-6} = 2.1 + 0.03 \times (\text{height});$$

where height is measured in inches.

This coefficient for height in this model is interpreted as, "each one-inch greater height is associated with, on average, a 0.03 pg/ml higher serum IL-6 level." However, the observed association between height and IL-6 levels could be confounded of by sex, because biological sex is linked with height and may also be associated with IL-6 levels. The possibility of confounding by sex can be investigated by adding a term for this characteristic to the multiple regression model:

$$\text{Mean IL-6} = \beta_0 + \beta_1 \times (\text{height}) + \beta_2 \times (\text{sex});$$

where sex is coded as 1 for men and 0 for women.

Solving this regression equation for the best fitting coefficients yields the following model:

$$\text{Mean IL-6} = 2.5 - 0.05 \times (\text{height}) + 0.7 \times (\text{sex})$$

Adding a variable for sex to the multiple regression model is equivalent to adjusting for this characteristic (by holding it constant). Before adjustment, each 1-inch greater height is associated with a 0.03 pg/ml *higher* serum IL-6 level. After adjustment for sex, each 1-inch greater height is associated with a −0.05 *lower* IL-6 level.

Recall from Chap. 10 that confounding is likely to be present if the size of an association changes meaningfully after adjustment for a potential confounding characteristic. The mathematical equivalent is to examine whether a *coefficient of interest* changes meaningfully after including the potential confounding characteristic in a multiple regression model. As previously described, there is no consensus rule as to how much change in the size of an association in response to adjustment constitutes a "meaningful" change. In this example, the coefficient for height changed from positive to negative, reversing the interpretation of the results and therefore indicating a meaningful change. These results are shown graphically in Fig. 16.11. Note that greater height is associated with lower IL-6 levels among both men and women, further demonstrating the confounding influence of sex in this example.

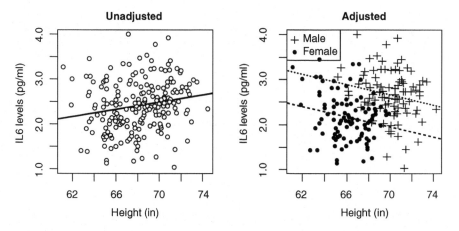

Fig. 16.11 Unadjusted and adjusted associations of height with interleukin-6 levels

16.5.2   Effect Modification

What about the possibility that the size of the association between height and IL-6 levels may differ between men and women? The standard multiple regression model would *not* be able to detect such a distinction, because the model includes only a single term, β_1 to define the association between height and IL-6 levels among all participants (men and women combined).

$$\text{Mean IL-6} = \beta_0 + \beta_1 \times (\text{height}) + \beta_2 \times (\text{sex});$$

where sex is coded as 1 for men and 0 for women.

A more complex model is needed to examine whether the size of the association between height and serum IL-6 levels may differ between men and women. Such a model would assume the form:

$$\text{Mean IL-6} = \beta_0 + \beta_1 \times (\text{height}) + \beta_2 \times (\text{sex}) + \beta_3 \times (\text{height} \times \text{sex})$$

The addition of the product term (height × sex) is needed to test for potential differences in the size of the association between height and serum IL-6 levels by sex (effect modification). Solving for the best fitting beta values yields the following regression equation:

$$\text{Mean IL-6} = -7.90 + 0.16 \times (\text{height}) + 17.2 \times (\text{sex}) - 0.25 \times (\text{height} \times \text{sex})$$

By design, this model is able to report different associations of height with IL-6 levels by sex. The association of height with IL-6 levels among women would be:

$$\text{Mean IL-6} = -7.90 + 0.16 \times (\text{height}) + 17.2 \times (0) - 0.25 \times (\text{height} \times 0)$$
$$= -7.90 + 0.16 \times (\text{height})$$

The results of this model would be interpreted as, "each one-inch greater height is associated with a 0.16 pg/ml higher IL-6 level, on average, among women."

The association of height with IL-6 levels among men would be:

$$\text{Mean IL-6} = -7.90 + 0.16 \times (\text{height}) + 17.2 \times (1) - 0.25 \times (\text{height} \times 1)$$
$$= -7.90 + 0.16 \times (\text{height}) - 0.25 \times (\text{height}) + 17.2$$
$$= -7.90 - 0.09 \times (\text{height}) + 17.2$$

The results of this model would be interpreted as, "each one-inch greater height is associated with a 0.09 pg/ml lower IL-6 level, on average, among men."

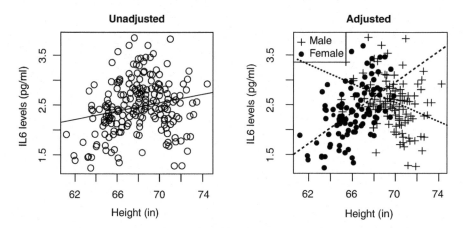

Fig. 16.12 Association of height with IL-6 levels; effect modification by sex

In this contrived example, the association between height and IL-6 levels *is modified by sex*, meaning that the size of the association differs meaningfully for women (slope = +0.16) compared to men (slope = −0.09). The coefficient for the interaction term (height × sex) represents the difference between the slopes relating height with IL-6 levels, shown in Fig. 16.12.

Chapter 17
Log-Link and Logistic Regression

Summary of Learning Points

17.1 Regression with log-link is useful for studying the relative change in an outcome variable.

    17.1.1 The log-link regression equation is described by: Log $[Y] = \beta_0 + \beta_1 \times (X)$.

    17.1.2 The antilog of each coefficient in a log-link model describes the relative difference in the outcome associated with a one-unit difference in the predictor variable.

17.2 Logistic regression is useful for studying associations of binary outcome variables.

    17.2.1 The antilog of each coefficient in a logistic regression model describes the odds ratio of the outcome associated with a one-unit difference in the predictor variable.

    17.2.2 For log-link and logistic regression models, the null hypothesis for a predictor variable is that the antilog of the coefficient equals 1.0.

17.1 Regression for Ratios

17.1.1 Log-Link Regression

The previous chapter described linear regression models, which assume the general form:

$$\text{Mean}(\text{outcome}) = \beta_0 + \beta_1 \times (\text{predictor} 1) + \beta_2 \times (\text{predictor} 2) + \beta_3 \times (\text{predictor} 3)\ldots$$

By definition, linear regression models specify a linear relationship between the predictor variables in the model and the outcome variable under study. In linear

© Springer Nature Switzerland AG 2019
B. Kestenbaum, *Epidemiology and Biostatistics*,
https://doi.org/10.1007/978-3-319-96644-1_17

regression, each one-unit difference in a predictor variable is associated with some constant difference in the mean value of the outcome variable. In many instances, the assumption of a linear relationship between two characteristics is reasonable. However, there are circumstances in which nonlinear relationships might be expected. For example, the HIV viral load, a measure of disease severity, grows exponentially over time among untreated patients, such that each week the viral load may be 10% greater than it was the previous week. This growth pattern motivates evaluation of the *relative change* (or percent change) in the HIV viral load.

A regression model that can be used to study the relative change in an outcome variable is called *regression with log-link* or *Poisson regression*. The log-link model assumes the following form:

$$Log(\text{mean outcome}) = \beta_0 + \beta_1 \times (\text{predictor 1}) + \beta_2 \times (\text{predictor 2}) \\ + \beta_3 \times (\text{predictor 3})\ldots$$

This model is identical to the linear regression model except for the addition of the log-term on the left-hand side of the equation. Consider the following log-link regression model to investigate age, HIV viral subtype, and coinfection with hepatitis C as potential risk factors for the severity of HIV infection, measured by the HIV viral load:

$$Log(\text{mean HIV viral load}) = \beta_0 + \beta_1 \times (\text{age}) + \beta_2 \times (\text{HIV subtype}) + \beta_3 \times (\text{hepatitis C});$$

where HIV subtype is coded as 1 for viral subtype D and 0 for all other subtypes and hepatitis C status is coded as 1 if hepatitis C is present and 0 if absent.

Using a computer to minimize the sum of squared residuals yields the following fitted equation:

$$Log(\text{mean HIV viral load}) = 9.4 + 0.08 \times (\text{age}) + 0.5 \times (\text{HIV subtype}) \\ + 0.3 \times (\text{hepatitis C})$$

In other words, coefficients of 0.08 for age, 0.5 for HIV subtype, 0.3 for hepatitis C, and 9.4 for the intercept yield the best fitting log-equation to the observed study data.

17.1.2 Interpretation of Log-Link Regression Models

The fitted log-link model can be used to answer the question, "what is the association of hepatitis C viral infection with the relative difference in HIV viral load, holding age, and HIV subtype constant?"

From the model, the log of the mean HIV viral load for *any* hepatitis C positive person in the study is:

$$Log(\text{mean HIV viral load}) = 9.4 + 0.08 \times (\text{age}) + 0.5 \times (\text{HIV subtype}) + 0.3 \times (1)$$

Analogously, the log of the mean HIV viral load for *any* hepatitis C negative person in the study is:

$$\mathrm{Log}(\text{mean HIV viral load}) = 9.4 + 0.08 \times (\text{age}) + 0.5 \times (\text{HIV subtype}) + 0.3 \times (0)$$

The difference in the log (mean HIV viral load), comparing people who are hepatitis C positive with those who are hepatitis C negative, holding age, and HIV subtype constant is:

$$\mathrm{Log}(\text{mean HIV viral load})_{\text{hepatitis C positive}} - \mathrm{Log}(\text{mean HIV viral load})_{\text{hepatitis C negative}}$$
$$= 9.4 + 0.08 \times (\text{age}) + 0.5 \times (\text{subtype}) + 0.3 \times (1) - 9.4 + 0.08 \times (\text{age})$$
$$+ 0.5 \times (\text{subtype}) + 0.3 \times (0)$$
$$= 0.3$$

All of the model terms cancel out except the coefficient for hepatitis C. Analogous to the linear regression model, the coefficient for any predictor variable in a log-link model represents the difference in the log (mean outcome) associated with each one-unit change in the predictor variable. Yet, the difference in the log (mean) value of an outcome variable is not easily interpretable. To decipher the results from the log-link model, a mathematical property of logarithms is needed.

For any two numerical values, *a* and *b*, it can be shown that: log *a* − log *b* = log (*a/b*). Therefore, the results from our log-link model:

$$\mathrm{Log}(\text{mean HIV viral load})_{\text{hepatitis C positive}} - \mathrm{Log}(\text{mean HIV viral load})_{\text{hepatitis C negative}} = 0.3$$

can be rewritten as:

$$\mathrm{Log}\left\{ \frac{\text{mean HIV viral load}_{\text{hepatitis C positive}}}{\text{mean HIV viral load}_{\text{hepatitis C negative}}} \right\} = 0.3$$

The next step is to take the antilog of both sides of the equation (exponentiate):

$$\mathrm{Exp}\left[\log\left\{ \frac{\text{mean HIV viral load}_{\text{hepatitis C positive}}}{\text{mean HIV viral load}_{\text{hepatitis C negative}}} \right\} \right] = \mathrm{Exp}[0.3]$$

which simplifies to:

$$\frac{\text{mean HIV viral load}_{\text{hepatitis C positive}}}{\text{mean HIV viral load}_{\text{hepatitis C negative}}} = \mathrm{Exp}[0.3]$$

Since the natural log (ln) is typically used in these models, the antilog is base e. Therefore,

$$\frac{\text{mean HIV viral load}_{\text{hepatitis C positive}}}{\text{mean HIV viral load}_{\text{hepatitis C negative}}} = \mathrm{Exp}[0.3] = 1.35$$

The interpretation of this result is that HIV viral load is, on average, *35% higher* for people who have hepatitis C infection, compared with people who do not have this infection, holding age, and HIV subtype constant. Stated another way, hepatitis C infection is associated with a 1.35-times higher HIV viral load, after adjustment for age and HIV subtype.

This example demonstrates that the antilog of each coefficient in a log-link regression model describes the relative difference in the outcome variable associated with each one-unit difference in the predictor variable.

Applying this interpretation to the coefficient for age in the log-link model: each 1-year-older age is associated with an exp (0.08) = 1.08-times higher, or 8% higher, HIV viral load, holding HIV subtype, and hepatitis C status constant.

Another useful application of evaluating study outcomes on the relative, rather than absolute scale is to facilitate comparison of associations between a risk factor of interest and a set of potentially interrelated outcome characteristics.

Example 17.1 High density lipoprotein cholesterol (HDL-C) particles are circulating assemblies of lipids and proteins that regulate key lipid metabolism pathways. The composition of HDL-C particles may be altered by vigorous physical activity. To pursue this hypothesis, researchers obtained end-of-study blood samples from a previously completed clinical trial, in which participants were randomly assigned to either an intensive 6-week exercise program or no prescribed exercise. The researchers examined the impact of the exercise program on three different HDL-C associated peptides.

First consider three fitted *linear* regression models to assess the effect of the exercise program on each HDL-C peptide:

$$\text{Model 1. Mean } (\text{peptide 1}) = 97 + 6.4 \times (\text{exercise})$$
$$\text{Model 2. Mean } (\text{peptide 2}) = 11 + 0.6 \times (\text{exercise})$$
$$\text{Model 3. Mean } (\text{peptide 3}) = 31 + 2.7 \times (\text{exercise})$$

where exercise is coded as 1 if the participant was assigned to exercise and 0 if they were assigned to no exercise.

The coefficients from these models suggest that exercise has the largest impact on peptide one. Specifically, the exercise program is associated with a 6.4-unit higher value of peptide 1, a 0.6-unit higher value of peptide 2, and a 2.7-unit higher value of peptide 3. However, this comparison assumes a similar meaning of one a unit difference in each HDL-C associated peptide. The total concentrations of peptides one, two, and three may differ dramatically, complicating the interpretation of differences expressed on an absolute scale.

Consider three fitted log-link regression models for the same study data:

$$\text{Model 1. } \text{Log} \left[\text{mean(peptide 1)} \right] = 97 + 0.1 \times (\text{exercise})$$
$$\text{Model 2. } \text{Log} \left[\text{mean(peptide 2)} \right] = 11 + 0.4 \times (\text{exercise})$$
$$\text{Model 3. } \text{Log} \left[\text{mean(peptide 3)} \right] = 31 + 0.5 \times (\text{exercise})$$

The log-link model expresses associations of the exercise program with the relative or percent difference in each peptide, facilitating comparison of the associations by converting them to the same scale. The exercise program is associated with an exp $(0.1) = 1.1$, or 10% higher value of peptide one, an exp $(0.4) = 1.5$, or 50% higher value of peptide two, and an exp $(0.5) = 1.6$, or 60% higher value of peptide three.

Note that negative coefficients in a log-link model indicate an association between a covariate and a relatively *lower* value of the outcome variable. For example, consider the following fitted log-link model for a hypothetical HDL-C peptide four:

$$\mathrm{Log}\big[\,\mathrm{mean}\,(\mathrm{peptide}\,4)\big] = 31 - 0.5 \times (\mathrm{exercise})$$

Based on the results of this model, the exercise program is associated with an exp $(-0.5) = 0.6$, or a $(1.0{-}0.6) = 40\%$ *lower* value of peptide four.

17.1.3   Hypothesis Testing for Log-Link Regression Results

Recall that for predictor variables in a linear regression model, the null hypothesis is that the coefficient for that variable is equal to 0, implying no association between the predictor variable and the mean value of the outcome. For log-link regression, the null hypothesis for a predictor variable is that the *antilog of the coefficient for that variable equals 1.0*, indicating a ratio of 1.0, or no association with the relative difference in the outcome variable.

17.2   Logistic Regression

17.2.1   Definition and Interpretation of the Logistic Regression Model

Historically, binary outcome variables posed a problem for linear and log-link regression models, because the probability of a binary outcome is bounded between 0 and 1, yet linear and log-link models assume that the outcome variable can take on an infinite number of possible values.

A mathematical approach to overcome this problem is to model the *odds of the outcome variable* rather than the probability. Odds are mathematically related to probabilities but can take on any positive value, which simplifies their use in regression models.

Modeling the log odds of a study outcome creates a new model called *logistic regression*, which is commonly used to study binary outcomes in clinical research studies. The logistic regression model assumes the following form:

$$\mathrm{Log}\,(\mathrm{odds\ outcome}) = \beta_0 + \beta_1 \times (\mathrm{predictor}\,1) + \beta_2 \times (\mathrm{predictor}\,2) + \beta_3 \times (\mathrm{predictor}\,3)\ldots$$

Recall the definition of *odds* from Chap. 7:

$$\text{Odds} = p / (1-p);$$

where p represents the probability of a given outcome.

While mathematically accommodating; odds are not intuitive. The interpretation of odds is facilitated by the property that *odds closely approximate probability when the disease outcome is rare*. A rare disease signifies that its probability, p, is small, resulting in a denominator for odds that is close to 1.0.

$$\text{Odds} = p / (1-p) \approx p \ \text{ if } p \text{ is small}$$

Example 17.1 Researchers conduct a case-control study to evaluate risk factors for community-acquired pneumonia. They identify a group of case patients who were recently diagnosed with community-acquired pneumonia and a group of control individuals who do not have pneumonia. Cases and controls are selected on the basis of being less than 65 years old, non-smokers, and having no previous history of cancer. The researchers review medical records to determine previous diagnoses of diabetes and asthma.

Consider a fitted logistic regression model for the association of age, diabetes, and asthma with community-acquired pneumonia:

$$\text{Log odds pneumonia} = \beta_0 + 0.1 \times (\text{age}) + 0.3 \times (\text{diabetes}) + 0.9 \times (\text{asthma})$$

Based on this model what is the association of asthma with pneumonia, after adjustment for age and diabetes?

For any person in the study who has a diagnosis of asthma:

$$\text{Log odds pneumonia} = \beta_0 + 0.1 \times (\text{age}) + 0.3 \times (\text{diabetes}) + 0.9 \times (1)$$

For any person in the study who does not have an asthma diagnosis:

$$\text{Log odds pneumonia} = \beta_0 + 0.1 \times (\text{age}) + 0.3 \times (\text{diabetes}) + 0.9 \times (0)$$

Therefore, comparison of the log odds of pneumonia between people with and without asthma:

$$\text{Log odds pneumonia}_{\text{asthma}} - \text{Log odds pneumonia}_{\text{no asthma}} = 0.9$$

Based on the property of logs, this equation can be rewritten as:

$$\text{Log}\left\{ \frac{\text{odds pneumonia}_{\text{asthma}}}{\text{odds pneumonia}_{\text{no asthma}}} \right\} = 0.9$$

Taking the antilog of both sides of the equation (using natural logs) yields:

$$\frac{\text{Odds pneumonia}_{\text{asthma}}}{\text{Odds pneumonia}_{\text{no asthma}}} = \text{Exp}\{0.9\} = 2.5$$

This result can be interpreted as: "asthma is associated with a 2.5-times higher odds of community-acquired pneumonia after adjustment for age and diabetes."

In logistic regression, the antilog of each coefficient in the model represents the association between a one-unit difference in the predictor variable and the *odds ratio* of the outcome variable holding the other variables in the model constant.

If pneumonia is relatively uncommon in the underlying population, then the term *odds* can be replaced with the more easily understood term *risk* or *probability*, yielding a sentence that is much more interpretable. In this example, the underlying population is relatively young non-smokers with no previous history of cancer. The probability of community-acquired pneumonia is likely to be relatively low in such a population, permitting replacement of the term *odds* with the term *risk*. On the other hand, if pneumonia were common in the underlying population, then the interpretation of the results from the logistic regression model is less clear due to the nonintuitive scale of odds. Statistical advances have now made it possible to use log-link models directly to estimate relative risks for binary outcomes, rather than approximating the relative risk using odds ratios. Nonetheless, logistic regression continues to be a popular analytic strategy for evaluating binary outcome data.

Similar to log-link regression, the null hypothesis for any predictor variable in a logistic regression model is that the *antilog of the coefficient for that predictor variable equals 1.0*, indicating an odds ratio of 1.0, or no association between the predictor and the outcome.

17.2.2 Interpreting Logistic Regression Results from Research Articles

Table 17.1 reports the results of a study of potential risk factors for peptic ulcer disease.

Based on these results, what type of regression model was used in this analysis?

- Logistic regression was likely used, because the outcome of the study is binary (peptic ulcer disease; yes versus no) and because the study reports adjusted odds ratios.

What is the functional form of the regression model?

- $\text{Log}\left(\text{odds peptic ulcer disease}\right) = \beta_0 + \beta_1 \times \text{age} + \beta_2 \times \text{sex} + \beta_3 \times \text{smoke}$
  $+ \beta_4 \times \text{spicy food} + \beta_5 \times \text{income} + \beta_6 \times H.pylori$

Table 17.1 Association of potential risk factors with peptic ulcer disease

	Adjusted odds ratio	95% confidence interval	P-value
Age (per decade)	1.15	(1.10, 1.30)	0.001
Female	0.85	(0.68, 1.05)	0.143
Current smoking	1.40	(1.20, 1.75)	0.040
Spicy food consumption	2.25	(0.90, 3.90)	0.060
Income (per $100,000 increase)	1.03	(1.02, 1.04)	0.001
H. pylori	1.70	(1.50, 2.80)	0.020

Results are adjusted for all of the characteristics in the table

A computer was used to find the best fitting values of the beta coefficients, such that the final model has the lowest sum of squared residuals. Once the logistic model has been fit, the antilog of each coefficient can be interpreted as the adjusted odds ratio of peptic ulcer disease associated with each predictor variable holding the other model variables constant.

What is the interpretation of the result for *H. pylori*?

- "Positive *H. pylori* status is associated with a 70% greater odds of peptic ulcer disease, compared with negative *H. pylori* status, after adjustment for age, sex, smoking, spicy food consumption, and income."

What is the interpretation of the *p*-value for *H. pylori*?

- "If *H. pylori* status is not associated with peptic ulcer disease in the underlying population, then the chance of observing this adjusted odds ratio of 1.7, or a more extreme adjusted odds ratio, is 2%. This low p-value implies that *H. pylori* *is* likely to be associated with peptic ulcer disease in the population.

Chapter 18
Survival Analysis

Summary of Learning Points

18.1 Incidence provides a compact summary of outcomes that occur during a study, but do not describe *when* these outcomes occur over time.

18.2 The survivor function, $S(t)$, returns the probability of being free of the study outcome at a given time, t.

    18.2.1 $S(t)$ is typically presented graphically as a function of follow-up time.

    18.2.2 $S(t)$ can be used to describe survival at a specific time point and median survival.

    18.2.3 Median survival is the elapsed time in which 50% of study subjects have incurred the outcome.

    18.2.4 The logrank test compares entire survival curves among different groups.

18.3 The Kaplan-Meier method is used to estimate $S(t)$ in the presence of censoring.

    18.3.1 Survival analysis is typically used to describe the first occurrence of a binary study outcome.

    18.3.2 Censoring refers to leaving a study for any reason before incurring the outcome.

    18.3.3 $S(t) \approx$ (probability of survival until time t) × (probability of survival through time t)

    18.3.4 The Kaplan-Meier estimation method assumes that censored individuals are similar to those who remain in the study.

    18.3.5 Kaplan-Meier survival plots typically present unadjusted study data.

18.4 Cox's proportional hazard model

    18.4.1 Handles censoring among different groups

    18.4.2 Can adjust for multiple confounding characteristics simultaneously

    18.4.3 Yields a hazard ratio, which very closely parallels the relative risk

18.5 Hazard ratios represent an average relative risk over a specified period of follow-up time.

© Springer Nature Switzerland AG 2019
B. Kestenbaum, *Epidemiology and Biostatistics*,
https://doi.org/10.1007/978-3-319-96644-1_18

18.5.1 Summary hazard ratios are meaningful for studies in which the relative risk remains roughly constant throughout follow-up.

18.5.2 Studies in which the relative risk changes meaningfully over time should ideally present separate hazard ratios for the relevant time periods of interest.

18.1   Motivation for Survival Data

Measures of incidence are commonly used to compare the occurrence of study outcomes over time, such as in randomized trials and cohort studies. Incidence provides a compact summary of outcomes that occur in a study but lack sufficient detail regarding *when* the outcomes occurred and may have limited applicability to clinical care.

Example 18.1   Abdominal aortic aneurysm (AAA) is a disease in which the lower portion of the aorta gradually dilates. The major risk of AAA is spontaneous rupture, which is often life threatening; however elective surgical repair can also be risky. Consider a 64-year-old man who is found to have a 5.0 cm AAA during routine ultrasound testing. He asks the following questions about his condition:

1. If I decide to have elective surgery, what is the chance that I will die within 5 years?
2. If I decide to have elective surgery, about how long can I expect to live?
3. If I survive the surgery, would my long-term survival be better than if I just waited?

To address the prognosis of small AAAs and to compare elective surgery versus routine medical care, the UK Small Aneurysm Trial randomly assigned 1029 patients who had an AAA <5.5 cm in diameter to either immediate surgical repair or close medical follow-up [1]. Trial participants were followed for more than 8 years for the primary outcome of all-cause mortality. The findings are presented in Table 18.1.

The incidence rate of all-cause mortality was equal between the early surgery and medical surveillance groups. These incidence data provide a compact summary of the deaths that occurred during the trial but do not directly answer the questions posed by the hypothetical patient who was diagnosed with a 5.0 cm AAA.

A second limitation of incidence measures is the possibility for bias under certain patterns of participant dropout. Consider the possibility that some participants

Table 18.1   Incidence of all-cause mortality in the UK Small Aneurysm Trial

	Number of people	Number of deaths	Person-years	Incidence proportion	Incidence rate[a]
Surgical group	563	242	3660	43.0%	6.6
Surveillance group	527	254	3820	48.2%	6.6

[a]Incidence rates expressed as deaths per 100 person-years

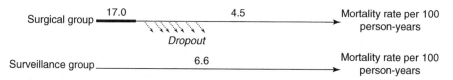

Fig. 18.1 Premature dropout of participants in the surgical group after completing surgery

in the surgical arm of the trial decide to leave the study after having successful surgery (these participants may no longer perceive any direct benefit from participation). Given the seriousness of AAA surgery, mortality is likely to be relatively high during the perioperative period and relatively low thereafter. Preferential dropout of participants in the surgical group after successful completion of surgery will delete the relatively low-risk postoperative time, when the benefits of surgery may be most pronounced. This specific pattern of dropout could artificially inflate the mortality *rate* in the surgical group and distort the comparison with the surveillance group, shown in Fig. 18.1.

18.2   Interpretation of Survival Data

18.2.1   Description of the Survivor Function

An alternative approach to reporting the AAA trial data is to describe the occurrence of mortality continuously throughout follow-up. This can be accomplished using the *survivor function*, which is denoted by the term $S(t)$. The survivor function is a function fit to the study data that returns the *cumulative probability of being free of the outcome at a particular time, t*. For the AAA study, the outcome is all-cause mortality; therefore, $S(t)$ represents the probability of being alive at time t. For example, let's say that $S(t)$ for the surgical arm of the AAA trial is defined by the equation:

$$S(t) = 1/(t+1);$$

where *t* represents years of follow-up.

The chance of surviving for 2 years in the surgical group would be $S(t) = 1/(1 + 2) = 0.33$ or 33%. We will explore how to obtain the survivor function shortly. For now, imagine that it has been handed to you for interpretation. Because the survivor function returns the continuous probability of being free of the study outcome, it is convenient to view $S(t)$ graphically as a function of follow-up time, shown in Fig. 18.2.

Compared to an incidence rate of 6.6 deaths per 100 person-years, the survivor function provides a much more descriptive account of survival in the surgical group. Because $S(t)$ is typically estimated using a method developed by Kaplan and Meier, survivor function plots are also called *Kaplan-Meier plots*.

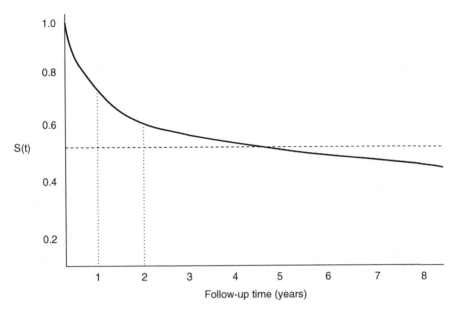

Fig. 18.2 Plot of hypothetical survivor function for the surgical group in the AAA trial.

18.2.2   Estimating Time-Specific and Median Survival from S(t)

To estimate survival at any particular time, a *vertical line* is drawn from the time point of interest to the survivor function. For example, a vertical line placed at 1 year on the *x*-axis of Fig 18.2 returns a 1-year survival probability of about 75% (dashed vertical line on the figure). The same procedure would estimate the 2-year survival probability to be about 60%. The survival plot answers relevant questions such as, "if a person with a small AAA decides to undergo elective surgery, what is the chance that they will be alive after 2 years?"

Median survival is defined as the elapsed time in which exactly 50% of the people in a treatment group or cohort have incurred the outcome. Median survival is estimated by drawing a *horizontal line* from the *y*-axis value of 0.5 to *S(t)* and then observing the associated follow-up time on the *x*-axis. For the survival plot in Fig. 18.2, median survival is about 4.5 years, depicted by the dashed horizontal line. Median survival can be estimated only from studies in which at least 50% of participants incur the outcome of interest.

Survival data for the nonsurgical group can be overlaid with that of the surgical group to compare relative differences in survival over time, depicted in Fig. 18.3.

The numbers presented underneath each year of the survival plot denote the number of participants in each group who remain in the study and free of the outcome. In this example, survival is initially higher among patients assigned to medical surveillance (dashed line) until about 3 years of follow-up, after which time

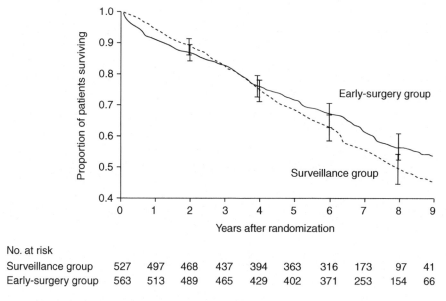

No. at risk

Surveillance group	527	497	468	437	394	363	316	173	97	41
Early-surgery group	563	513	489	465	429	402	371	253	154	66

Fig. 18.3   Survival in UK Small Aneurysm Trial

survival is higher in the surgery group (solid line). Note that it is *not* possible to *compare* median survival in this example because the surgical group does not quite reach 50% survival.

18.2.3   Statistical Testing of Survival Data

The superimposed survival curves may prompt the question, "is survival significantly different between the two groups at a given time?" For example, the data in Fig. 18.3 reveal that survival at 8 years is about 57% in the surgical group and about 50% in the surveillance group. Are these two survival probabilities statistically different? Recall that the chi-square test is used to test proportions between two different groups. Testing the proportions obtained from survival data requires more complex statistical methods, but the interpretation of p-values obtained from these tests is similar. A statistical test of 8-year survival between the surgical and surveillance groups yields a p-value of 0.05. The interpretation of this p-value is, "if there is truly no difference in 8-year survival, comparing early surgery to surveillance in the population of all similar patients with a small AAA, then the chance of observing this 7% difference in 8-year survival, or a more extreme difference, is 5%." The results of statistical inference testing imply that observing this difference in 8-year survival would be unlikely if 8-year survival was truly equal in the population.

The 95% confidence interval for the difference in 8-year survival, comparing surgery to surveillance, is: 1% higher - 13% higher. This confidence interval can be interpreted as, "there is '95% confidence' that the difference in 8-year survival, comparing surgery to surveillance could be as little as 1% higher or as great as 13% higher in the underlying population of similar AAA patients."

Limitations of statistical testing of the survivor function are analogous to previously discussed concerns regarding statistical testing.

- Problems of multiple comparisons may arise from testing survival at too many specific times, such as 1-year, 2-year, and 3-year survival, because multiple testing will increase the possibility of observing a false-positive association. Methods to account for multiple comparisons can be used to address this problem by setting a more stringent threshold for defining a significant p-value.
- Attrition during follow-up markedly diminishes statistical power for detecting long-term differences in survival. For the AAA trial, only 97 participants in the surveillance group and 154 participants in the surgical group, remained alive and in the study after 8 years of follow-up.

Another statistical question motivated by the superimposed survival data might be, "are the two survival curves significantly different overall?" This question is usually addressed by a statistical test called the *logrank test*, although other tests have been developed for this purpose. The logrank test compares *entire survival curves* among different treatment groups. The p-value from the logrank test represents the probability of obtaining the observed difference in survival curves, or more extremely different survival curves, if these curves are in fact the same in the population. Applying the logrank test to the AAA study data returns of a p-value of 0.05. The interpretation of this p-value is, "if survival curves for the surgery and surveillance groups were identical in the underlying population, then the chance of observing these different survival curves, or more extremely different survival curves is 5%."

However, the logrank test is not particularly useful for the AAA trial data, because the survival curves for the surgery and surveillance groups cross. Results from the logrank test demonstrate only that the two survival curves are likely to be different from each other in the population. The more complete story is that survival was initially better in the surveillance group and then subsequently better in the surgical group later in the study. The logrank test is most useful for studies in which the survival curves remain separated throughout follow-up. For such studies, a statistically significant result from the logrank test implies that *overall survival* in one group is statistically better (or worse) than *overall survival* in the other group.

18.3 Estimation of the Survivor Function

18.3.1 Definitions of Outcomes and Censoring

Survival analysis evaluates the probability of a *binary outcome*, also called an *event*, or a *failure*. In most instances, survival analysis is used to describe the first occurrence of an outcome in a study. Participants who incur the outcome of interest are considered to have completed the study at that time and are typically no longer followed. This strategy may seem obvious for mortality outcomes but applies similarly to studies of nonfatal events. For example, a clinical trial compared the impact of two cardiac rehabilitation programs on the risk of heart failure. Participants in this study were followed until they either developed heart failure, left the study prematurely, or the study ended, whichever came first.

In survival analysis, the first occurrence of an outcome refers to the first occurrence during the study period, regardless of whether the outcome previously occurred during a person's lifetime. In the heart failure study, the first occurrence of heart failure could represent incident disease if the participant had no previous history of heart failure at the start of the study, or recurrent disease if they had a previous diagnosis of heart failure at entry. From a survival analysis perspective, both studies are the same in that they assess the probability of heart failure-free survival over the course of the study. More advanced survival analysis techniques are available for studying multiple events per participant in a study but are beyond the scope of this book.

The most accurate estimate of $S(t)$ is obtained when every person in a study is followed until they develop the outcome of interest. However, clinical studies rarely, if ever, obtain complete follow-up data because (1) participants drop out or are lost to follow-up before incurring the outcome of interest, (2) studies end at some predetermined time, or (3) death occurs in studies of nonfatal outcomes. *Censoring* is defined as *leaving a study for any reason other than incurring the outcome of interest*. For example, participants in the AAA study were censored if they dropped out, were lost to follow-up, or were still alive when the study was terminated after 10 years as planned. For studies of nonfatal outcomes, participants are also censored at the time of death, because in such studies death is equivalent to leaving the study before incurring the outcome of interest. Similarly, for studies that evaluate specific causes of death, such as cancer mortality, participants are censored at the time of death due to other causes. Censoring results in having some information about a person's survival time, but not knowing their survival time exactly.

18.3.2   *Kaplan-Meier Estimation of the Survivor Function for Uncensored Data*

In practice $S(t)$ is *estimated* using the study data. The most direct way to estimate $S(t)$ from the AAA study data would be to check on the survival status of the study population as often as possible. For example, survival status of 10 hypothetical participants in the AAA study could be updated every day, shown in Table 18.2.

$S(t)$ represents the probability of survival *after* the specified follow-up time has elapsed. For example, $S(6 \text{ days}) = 0.6$, indicating that there is a 60% chance of survival *after* 6 days of follow-up in this group of 10 participants. It is important to note that $S(t)$ *changes only when the study outcome occurs*. Intervals of follow-up time without events have the same $S(t)$ value as the previous period. Therefore, survival data can be presented in a more compact form, shown in Table 18.3.

Table 18.2 Survival status for 10 hypothetical participants in the small aneurysm trial

Follow-up time	Number of people at risk	Events (deaths)	$S(t)$
1 day	10	0	1.0
2 days	10	1	0.9
3 days	9	1	0.8
4 days	8	0	0.8
5 days	8	0	0.8
6 days	8	2	0.6
7 days	6	0	0.6
8 days	6	2	0.4

Table 18.3 Compact presentation of survival data

Follow-up time	Number of people at risk	Events (deaths)	$S(t)$
2 days	10	1	0.9
3 days	9	1	0.8
6 days	8	2	0.6
8 days	6	2	0.4

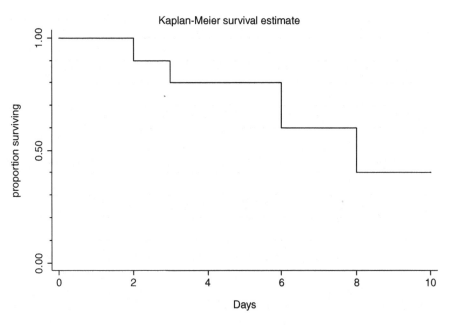

Fig. 18.4 Estimate of the survivor function for 10 hypothetical study participants

These data reveal that $S(t)$ is not a smooth, continuous curve, but rather a step function, with the "steps" occurring at the failure times. Figure 18.4 plots $S(t)$ as a function of time for the group of 10 hypothetical study participants.

18.3.3   Kaplan-Meier Estimation of the Survivor Function for Censored Data

The above example considered an idealized situation, in which participants were assumed to have remained in the study throughout the 10-day period of interest. In real-life situations, $S(t)$ must be estimated in the presence of censoring, which is defined as leaving a study for any reason other than incurring the outcome of interest. Table 18.4 adds censoring information to the original survival data.

How is $S(t)$ calculated for day 5, when two participants drop out of the study? Because $S(t)$ changes only when study outcomes occur, $S(t)$ for day 5 will remain 0.8, despite the loss of these two participants. However, removal of these two participants will decrease the number of people who are risk for the outcome at the start of the next time interval on day 6.

How is $S(t)$ calculated for day 6? Unfortunately, the survival status of the two participants who dropped out is no longer known. If these two participants died during day 6, then $S(t)$ at the end of day 6 would be 0.4. On the other hand, if these two participants survived through day 6, then $S(t)$ at the end of day 6 would be 0.6. Censoring prevents knowing the exact value of $S(t)$.

The solution to this problem is to estimate $S(t)$ from the product of two probabilities:

$$S(t) = (\text{probability of survival until time } t) \times (\text{probability of survival through time } t)$$

The probability of survival until time t is simply $S(t)$ at the end of the previous time period. In other words, the probability of survival until day 6 is the probability of survival at the end of day 5, which is 0.8. The probability of survival through time t is calculated based on the number of people who remain in the study at the start of this time period. For day 6, there are six people who are alive at the beginning of the day, among whom, four remain alive at the end of the day.

Number of people at risk at start of day 6	Deaths occurring on day 6	Probability of death on day 6	Probability of survival on day 6
6	2	2/6 = 0.333	4/6 = 0.667

Table 18.4 Survival status for 10 hypothetical participants in the presence of censoring

Follow-up time	Subjects at risk	Events (deaths)	Dropouts	$S(t)$
1 day	10	0	0	1.0
2 days	10	1	0	0.9
3 days	9	1	0	0.8
4 days	8	0	0	0.8
5 days	8	0	2	?
6 days	6	2	1	?
7 days	3	0	0	?
8 days	3	2	0	?

$$S(\text{day } 6) = (\text{probability of survival until day } 6) \times (\text{probability of survival through day } 6)$$
$$= 0.8 \times (4/6) = 0.533$$

The calculation of S(t) for the end of day 7 remains 0.533, because of the important property that $S(t)$ remains constant in the absence of events. The next study outcome occurs on day 8. The probability of survival through day 8, given survival until day 8, is 1/3, because three people are alive at the start of day 8, and one survives. Therefore, the cumulative probability of survival past day 8 is $0.53 \times (1/3) = 0.18$. Table 18.5 and Fig. 18.5 present censored survival data for the 10 hypothetical study participants.

Table 18.5 Survival status for 10 hypothetical participants in the presence of censoring

Follow-up time	Subjects at risk	Events (deaths)	Dropouts	$S(t)$
1 day	10	0	0	1.0
2 days	10	1	0	0.9
3 days	9	1	0	0.8
4 days	8	0	0	0.8
5 days	8	0	2	0.8
6 days	6	2	1	0.8 × (4/6) = 0.53
7 days	3	0	0	0.53
8 days	3	2	0	0.53 × (1/3) = 0.18

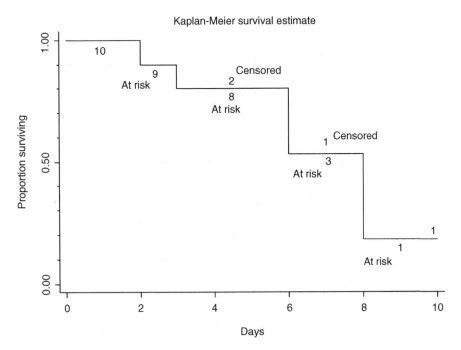

Fig. 18.5 Survival status for 10 hypothetical participants in presence of censoring

This common approach for estimating $S(t)$ in the presence of censoring is called the *Kaplan-Meier* or *product-limit method*. The Kaplan-Meier method allows people to contribute information to $S(t)$ as long as they remain in a study and then stop contributing information when their data are censored. For the two participants who dropped out of the study on day 5, the Kaplan-Meier method used their data for the first 5 study days and then removed them from the analysis by reducing the number of at-risk individuals for the next calculation of $S(t)$.

An inherent assumption of survival data obtained using the Kaplan-Meier method is that censored individuals are similar to those who remain in the study, an assumption known as "non-informative" censoring. This assumption is likely to hold if participants are censored for reasons unlikely to be related to the study outcome, for example, if people drop out of a study due to relocation or the study ends at a predetermined time. In other instances, the assumption of non-informative censoring may be less certain, for example, if participants leave a study after experiencing a severe adverse event caused by a study treatment.

The Kaplan-Meier method estimates $S(t)$ based on the timing of the study outcomes and the pattern of censoring. However, survival data are *not* typically adjusted for potential differences in participant characteristics that may exist among treatment or exposure groups. Consequently, Kaplan-Meier plots have a relatively straightforward interpretation for large randomized trials, in which participant characteristics are likely to be similar across treatment and control groups but have less certain interpretation for observational data. Imagine that the AAA study data were collected from an observational cohort study that compared survival of patients who underwent elective AAA surgery to that of patients who did not undergo surgery? In the observational study, patients who undergo surgery may differ from patients who are followed medically, in terms of age, comorbidity, and other characteristics. The Kaplan-Meier plot would present the raw, unadjusted study data, which may be confounded.

18.4 Cox's Proportional Hazards Model

For studies of outcomes over time in which confounding is of particular concern, methods are needed to handle censoring *and* adjust for potential differences in participant characteristics. A solution to this problem was first published by Cox in 1972. His proportional hazards model remains the most widely used method for analyzing survival data in clinical and epidemiological research, because it elegantly handles censoring and permits simultaneous adjustment for multiple confounding characteristics. The following is an oversimplified description of how the proportional hazards model works.

Recall from Chap. 17 that logistic regression is used to model the log odds ratio of a binary outcome variable as a function of predictor covariates:

$$\log \text{odds}\, Y = \beta_0 + \beta_1 \times (\text{treatment}) \dots$$

The logistic regression model does not inherently account for follow-up time. Differences in person-time among the treatment or exposure groups could lead to erroneous results. One solution is to add a term for follow-up time to the logistic regression model:

$$\log \text{odds } Y = \beta_0 + \beta_1 \times (\text{treatment}) + \beta_2 \times (\text{follow-up time}) \ldots$$

However, this model assumes a linear relationship between the log odds of the outcome and follow-up time. In reality, the exact nature of the relationship between the study outcome and person-time is typically unknown. Moreover, differential censoring could still lead to bias in this model, which simply counts person-time in each group.

The Cox model exploits the important property demonstrated by the Kaplan-Meier estimation method that information about survival is obtained only when a study outome occurs. The Cox model essentially performs logistic-like regression repeatedly at every failure time in a study. This procedure assures that follow-up time is always identical for all participants at the time of each comparison. Figure 18.6 presents a simplified diagram of the proportion hazards model approach for the first 10 hypothetical participants in the AAA study.

For the first event (death), occurring on study day 2, a fully adjusted logistic-like regression model is fit to predict the association between treatment (surgery versus surveillance) and mortality, holding the other variables in the model constant. The model is fit for the single death occurring on day 2, ensuring that follow-up time is the same for everyone in the model, but yielding wildly variable estimates based on only a single outcome. The identical model is then fit again for the second event, occurring on day 3, and the results from this model are averaged with those of the first model. Subsequent models are then fit for events occurring on days six and eight, and for every subsequent event during follow-up. The results from all of these models are averaged together to produce a summary result. As more events are added, estimates for the variables in the model stabilize, with progressively lower variation.

The important fact to notice is that each model holds follow-up time constant by comparing participants who have been in the study for the same amount of time. For

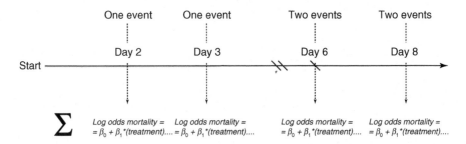

Fig. 18.6 Simplified description of Cox's proportional hazards model

the first model, all participants under comparison have been in the study for exactly 2 days. For the second model, all participants have been in the study for exactly 3 days. This procedure is analogous to matching on follow-up time, thereby accounting for differences in risk time among the treatment groups.

What about censoring? Like the Kaplan-Meier method for estimating $S(t)$, the Cox model ignores participants who leave a study in between events but removes them from subsequent analyses at the time of the next event. The two people who dropped out of the study on day 5 (diagonal lines in the figure) will contribute data to the first two models on days 2 and 3, but will not contribute data to any subsequent models. In this way, the analyses are performed among only people who are at risk for the outcome.

The Cox model yields a measure of risk called the *hazard ratio*, which very closely parallels relative risk. Recall that logistic regression is used to model the odds ratio of disease and that the odds ratio approximates the relative risk when the prevalence of disease is low. The Cox model makes use of this property by keeping the prevalence of disease very low for each comparison, because only one or a small number of events are expected at any given follow-up time. By fitting separate logistic models for each failure time, the Cox model ensures that the prevalence of the outcome will be low for each model.

18.5   Interpreting Survival Data

18.5.1   Interpreting Hazard Ratios

Hazard ratios are calculated by averaging the results of models fit across some period of follow-up time, often the entire study period. Consequently, hazard ratios represent *summary relative risks* during follow-up. Consider the primary results published from the AAA study:

	Adjusted hazard ratio (95% confidence interval)
Surgery (versus surveillance)	0.83 (0.69, 1.00)

The term "hazard ratio" implies that the result was obtained from a proportional hazards model. This summary hazard ratio was obtained by averaging the instantaneous hazard ratios of mortality over the entire duration of the study. The value of 0.83 can be interpreted as, "the relative hazard of mortality is 17% lower among participants who were assigned to surgery, compared with those assigned to surveillance, accounting for potential differences in follow-up time between the treatment groups." The similarity between the hazard ratio and the relative risk permit replacement of the term "hazard" with the term "risk" for a more straightforward interpretation.

A summary hazard ratio is meaningful for studies in which the relative risk remains roughly constant throughout follow-up. For example, a clinical trial comparing a new antiviral treatment to placebo among patients with hepatitis C found consistently higher hepatitis C-free survival in the active treatment group throughout the course of the study. The summary hazard ratio reported for this study therefore provides a reasonable description of the impact of antiviral treatment on this outcome.

On the other hand, summary hazard ratios can be misleading for studies in which the relative risk differs over time. In the UK Small Aneurysm Trial, early surgery was initially associated with lower survival than medical surveillance but was then associated with greater survival later in the study. The summary hazard ratio of 0.83 reported for this study oversimplifies the association of AAA surgery with mortality. A more complete way to present the trial results would be to calculate and show separate hazard ratios for the early and late study periods, shown in Table 18.6.

Computing separate hazard ratios for different follow-up periods provides a more complete picture of how surgical AAA repair impacts mortality. Surgery was associated with a 2.5 times higher risk of death compared with surveillance during the first 6 months of the trial, reflecting the high postoperative mortality associated with this procedure. From 6 months until the end of the study, surgery was associated with a $(1.0-0.77) = 23\%$ lower relative risk of death compared with surveillance, reflecting the relative benefit of surgery among people who survive the procedure. For studies in which the relative risk changes in a clinically important manner over follow-up, separate hazard ratios should ideally be reported for the relevant time periods of interest.

Some controversy may arise as to *how much difference* in relative risk over follow-up should prompt calculation and presentation of separate relative risks for shorter time periods and how many different follow-up periods should be presented. The stability of hazard ratios obtained from the Cox model increases with greater numbers of study outcomes. Splitting the data into too many small pieces can yield unreliable estimates and create problems of multiple comparisons. A statistical test of the proportional hazards assumption can be helpful for addressing this issue, by evaluating whether the relative risk is "significantly" different over the course of follow-up time. However, the decision to present separate hazard ratios should not depend solely on the results of statistical testing, but also on clinical or scientific knowledge of how the treatment or exposure is expected to impact the disease process over time.

Table 18.6 Hazard ratios for early and late study periods in the UK Small Aneurysm Trial	Adjusted hazard ratio (95% confidence interval)
Follow-up time 0–6 months	
Surgery (versus surveillance)	2.52 (1.20, 5.33)
Follow-up time > 6 months	
Surgery (versus surveillance)	0.77 (0.63, 0.93)

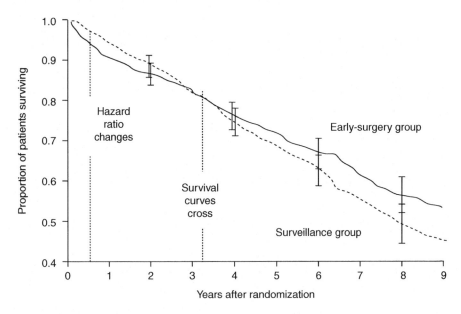

Fig. 18.7 Changes in hazard ratios and survival curves

18.5.2   Interpreting Survival Versus Hazard Ratio Data

Based on the data in Table 18.6, the hazard ratios in the UK Small Aneurysm Trial differed relatively quickly after surgery. However, the survival curves did not cross until after 3 years of follow-up, shown in Fig. 18.7.

This discrepancy reflects the natural relationship between $S(t)$ and the hazard ratio. The hazard ratio represents a ratio of *rates* at which the study outcome occurs over time, whereas $S(t)$ compares overall disease-free survival at that time. The markedly higher mortality *rate* in the surgical group during the first 6 months of trial translates into a greater absolute number of deaths during this period. This survival difference is documented by $S(t)$, which describes the proportion of people who remain alive in each group:

	Alive at start of study	Deaths during first 6 months	Alive after 6 months	S (6 months)
Surgical group	563	31	532	94.5%
Surveillance group	527	12	515	97.7%
		Hazard ratio = 2.5 comparing surgery to surveillance		

After 6 months, the hazard ratio indicates a lower relative *rate* of death in the surgical group, compared with that of the surveillance group. Yet, it takes another

2.5 years for this lower rate to translate into an equal proportion of people remaining alive in each group.

Survival data and hazard ratios are directly applicable to clinical decision-making and patient education. One perspective on the AAA trial data is that successful elective surgery translates fairly quickly into lower rates of death for people who can survive the surgery. Another perspective is that overall survival does not favor surgery until at least 3 years, such that people who may have a relatively short life expectancy due to extensive comorbidity may elect to avoid this surgery. Clinical studies frequently present Kaplan-Meier survival estimates *and* hazard ratios, because the combination of these measures provides the most complete picture of overall disease-free survival and rates of disease development.

Reference

1. United Kingdom Small Aneurysm Trial P, Powell JT, Brady AR, et al. Long-term outcomes of immediate repair compared with surveillance of small abdominal aortic aneurysms. N Engl J Med. 2002;346(19):1445–52.

Glossary of Terms

Adjustment	A process of isolating the effect of a single factor while holding differences in the composition of a population constant. Methods for adjustment include restriction, stratification, matching, regression and randomization
ANOVA test	A statistical test used to compare the mean value of a characteristic among multiple groups
Arithmetic mean	The expected value of a variable, defined as $\sum x_i / N$
Attributable risk *Risk difference* *Absolute risk* *reduction*	Incidence(exposed cohort) – Incidence(unexposed cohort) Describes the quantity of additional outcomes in the exposed group that is presumably due to the exposure
Attributable risk %	$$\frac{\left[\text{Incidence}\left(\text{exposed cohort}\right) - \text{Incidence}\left(\text{unexposed cohort}\right)\right] \times 100\%}{\text{Incidence}\left(\text{exposed cohort}\right)}$$
Bias toward the null *Conservative* *error*	Biases that lead to observing an attenuated measure of risk compared with the true impact of a risk factor or treatment
Binary variable *Dichotomous* *variable; event*	A variable that can take on only two possible values
Blinding	A procedure used in clinical trials to prevent participants from knowing which intervention they are receiving and investigators from knowing which interventions are administered throughout the trial
Block randomization	A restricted randomization strategy that performs randomization within smaller groups of participants. Must be planned prior to the implementation of a trial and incorporated into the randomization process
Bonferroni correction	A simple method to correct for the problem of multiple comparisons that limits the study-wide type I error rate to 5% by setting the p-value threshold for significance *at 0.05/the total number of tests*
Box plot	A graphical description of a single variable that includes a horizontal bar representing the median, a shaded region representing the 25th and 75th quantiles, and "whiskers" to 1.5 times the 25th and 75th quantiles. Extreme observations are displayed as open circles beyond the whiskers

© Springer Nature Switzerland AG 2019
B. Kestenbaum, *Epidemiology and Biostatistics*,
https://doi.org/10.1007/978-3-319-96644-1

C-statistic	A statistical measure used to describe the overall predictive capability of a continuous test. Values >0.8 indicate generally good overall prediction
Case-control study	A type of observational study that identifies people with and without a specific condition of interest and then works backward to determine the proportions who had a previous exposure
Case report	A type of observational study that describes the experience of a single person with a disease or condition
Case series	A type of observational study that describes the experience of a group of people with a disease or condition
Categorical variable *Ordinal variable* *Nominal variable*	A variable that can take on only a few possible values. Categorical variables can be further classified as *ordered* when possible responses correspond to a hierarchical scale (such as income categories) or nominal if there is no ordered distinction among the possible responses (such as race)
Causal inference	The appraisal of whether a potential risk factor is likely to be a cause of the disease. Criteria to assess causal inference include randomized studies, strong associations, temporal relationships, exposure varying associations, and biological plausibility
Causal pathway	A conceptual group of mechanisms that plausibly explain how the exposure of interest is presumed to influence the disease process
Censoring	Leaving a study for any reason other than incurring the outcome of interest, such as dropout, loss to follow-up, the predetermined end of a study, or death in studies of non-mortality outcomes
Chi-square test	A statistical test used to compare proportions between two or more groups
Clinical trial	An interventional study
Coefficient	The constants associated with the predictor variables in regression For the model: Mean $(Y) = \beta_0 + \beta_1 \times (X_1)$ β_1 is the *coefficient* for the predictor variable X_1 Individual coefficients from a multiple regression model represent the independent association between the predictor variable and the outcome variable, holding all other variables in the model constant
Coefficient of variation	(Standard deviation of test/mean value of test) × 100% Describes the reliability of a continuous test or measurement
Continuous variable	A variable that can take on an infinite number of possible values
Cohort	A group of people derived from a study population who share a common experience or condition and whose outcome is unknown at the beginning of the study
Cohort study	A type of observational study that compares the incidence of the disease outcome among different cohorts
Concealment	A procedure used in randomized trials that shields the personnel who assign the interventions from the identity of these interventions to ensure faithful random treatment allocation
Confidence interval (95%)	An interval placed around the result of an experiment such that 95% of all such intervals will contain the true result in the population
Confounding	A type of bias inherent in observational studies, in which characteristics other than the exposure of interest distort the observed association between exposure and disease

Confounding by indication	A type of confounding that may arise in observational studies of the consequences of medications or procedures
Confounding characteristic	A characteristic that is associated with the exposure, associated with the outcome, and does not reside on the causal pathway. Can also be identified by a meaningful change in the size of an association after adjustment
CONSORT	*Consolidated Standards of Reporting Trials* A checklist of standardized items used to facilitate the reporting of clinical trial results and simplify their interpretation
Continuous variable	A type of data that can take on a theoretically infinite number of possible values
Control procedures	Procedures administered as a comparator in clinical trials, such as a placebo, a similar treatment, delayed treatment, an accepted standard of care, or no treatment at all
Correlation	A summary measure that describes agreement between two continuous variables. A correlation coefficient of +1 indicates perfect positive agreement, a correlation coefficient of −1 indicates perfect negative agreement, and a correlation coefficient of 0 indicates no agreement
Cox proportional hazard model	A regression method for survival data that accounts for censoring and can adjust for multiple characteristics simultaneously
Cross-sectional study	A type of observational study in which the exposure and outcome are measured at the same time
Crossover trial	A type of clinical trial in which participants are randomly assigned to receive the study treatments in different orders
Crude measures of risk *Unadjusted measures*	Measures of risk, such as relative risk, odds ratio, or attributable risk, calculated using raw study data and not adjusted for potential differences in participant characteristics
Cutoff value *Cut point*	A value used to divide a continuous characteristic into two or more groups. May be used to define a positive versus negative test.
Diagnosis	Testing for disease during the clinical phase, in which symptoms and/or signs of the disease are present at the time of testing
Differential misclassification *Selective misclassification*	Measurement error that occurs systematically within a study – either error in exposure measurements that depend on the outcome or error in outcome measurements that depend on the exposure. Can have a wide range of impacts on the observed association, including exaggerating the association, diluting the association, or creating false associations
Double blind study	A study in which both the participants and the investigators are unaware of which interventions are administered
Effect modification *Interaction*	The size of an association differs by another characteristic
Effect size	The magnitude of an effect or association
Efficacy	The benefits and harms of an intervention assessed under ideal conditions
Effectiveness	The practical benefits and harms of an intervention assessed among diverse groups of people in realistic settings
Equipoise	The point in which a rational and informed person has no preference among two or more available treatments based on available knowledge

Exclusion criteria	Criteria applied to a source population to obtain the specific study population
External validity *Applicability*; *generalizability*	Addresses whether the results of a study are likely to be broadly applicable to other groups of people and environments. In the context of statistical inference, external validity is a subjective, not mathematical, term that describes whether a population is clinically or scientifically relevant
Exposure *Risk factor*; *predictor*	A characteristic that may explain or predict the presence of an outcome
Exposure-varying association	Greater amounts of a risk factor or exposure are associated with progressively higher risks of the disease
Factorial trial	A type of randomized trial in which participants receive combinations of treatments or control procedures in the same trial
Geometric mean	Geometric mean = $\exp \left[\sum \ln (x_i)/N \right]$ A measure of central tendency that is less influenced by outlying values than the arithmetic mean.
Gold standard	A procedure used to ascertain idealized study data. Gold-standard procedures are typically complex, invasive, and/or expensive
Hazard ratio	The summary relative risk over a given period of study time. Derived from a Cox proportional hazards model
Histogram	A summary measure for a single variable that plots observed values on the x-axis versus relative frequency of these values on the y-axis
Incidence	The rate of new disease development over a period of time
Incidence proportion *Cumulative incidence*	$\dfrac{\left(\text{Number of new cases of disease that develop over time} \right)}{\left(\text{Population without disease at baseline} \right)} \times 100\%$
Incidence rate *Incidence density*	$\dfrac{\text{Number of new cases of disease that develop over time}}{\text{Person} - \text{time at risk}}$
Influential point	A data point that meaningfully alters the slope of a regression equation. Influential points have extreme values on both the x- and y-axes
Intention-to treat analysis	Evaluates all participants who are initially randomized in a clinical trial according to their initial treatment assignments
Internal validity	The ability of a study to accurately answer the proposed research question within the given study population and environment
Interquartile range	The 25th and 75th quantiles (percentiles) of a distribution
Intervention	Any form of therapy, such as a drug, procedure, or lifestyle modification, that is administered in a clinical trial
Interventional study *Clinical trial*	A type of study design in which participants are assigned to one or more interventions or control procedures
Kaplan-Meier plot *Survival plot*	A plot of the survivor function on the y-axis versus follow-up time on the x-axis
Kaplan-Meier estimator *Product-limit method*	A method for estimating the survivor function in the presence of censoring $S(t) = (\text{survival probability until } t) \times (\text{survival probability past } t)$

Kappa statistic	Describes the proportion of binary tests that are in agreement between two observers beyond that expected from chance. Absolute Kappa statistic values >0.6 are considered to represent reasonably good agreement
Lead time bias	A type of bias that can occur in observational studies of screening in which additional follow-up time is preferentially added to the screened group, creating the appearance of a survival benefit
Length bias sampling *Length time bias*	A type of bias that can occur in observational studies of screening in which more slowly progressing variants of a disease are preferentially detected by a screening program
Likelihood ratio	Likelihood ratio positive = sensitivity/(1 − specificity) Likelihood ratio negative = (1 − sensitivity)/specificity Likelihood ratios combine sensitivity and specificity of a test to convert pretest probabilities into post-test probabilities using a nomogram
Linear regression	Regression using an equation that assumes the form: Mean $(Y) = \beta_0 + \beta_1 \times$ (predictor1) $+ \beta_2 \times$ (predictor2)… where Y is a continuous outcome variable
Log-link regression *Poisson regression*	Regression using an equation that assumes the form: Log (mean Y) $= \beta_0 + \beta_1 \times$ (predictor1) $+ \beta_2 \times$ (predictor2)… where Y is a continuous outcome variable
Logistic regression	Regression using an equation that assumes the form: Log (odds outcome) $= \beta_0 + \beta_1 \times$ (predictor1) $+ \beta_2 \times$ (predictor2)… where Y is a binary outcome variable
Logrank test	A statistical test that examines entire survival curves among different treatment groups. The p-value for the logrank test is the probability of obtaining the observed survival curves, or more extremely different survival curves, if the survival curves are in fact identical in the population
Matching	A procedure performed during the conduct of a study to increase the degree of similarity in participant characteristics among groups
Measures of disease frequency	Tools for quantifying the burden and occurrence of disease in populations
Measures of effect	Measures that compare the risks of disease among groups, such as relative risk, attributable risk, or population attributable risk
Median survival	The time point during follow-up in which exactly half of a study population has incurred the outcome
Median value	The value within a distribution for which exactly half of the data fall above this value and half fall below it
Mediator	A characteristic that represents a plausible mechanism by which the exposure of interest may influence the disease process. Mediators reside on the causal of pathway of association – they are not confounders
Misclassifica-tion *Information bias*	The false characterization of a study characteristic due to measurement error. May be non-differential of differential
Multiple comparisons	A problem that arises from performing multiple statistical hypothesis tests on the same study data, thereby increasing the chance of a type I error
Multiple regression	A statistical method used to adjust for several confounding characteristics simultaneously

Negative predictive value	$\dfrac{\text{Number with gold} - \text{standard absence of disease who test negative}}{\text{Number of people who test negative}}$ The probability of not having actual disease given a negative test.
Nested case-control study	A type of case-control study in which the cases and controls are selected from a larger unified population
Non-differential misclassification *Non-selective misclassification*	Misclassification that occurs randomly, or roughly equally across a study population. Typically causes a dilution of the observed relative risk compared to the true relative risk that would be obtained under idealized measurements
Normal distribution	A distribution for which the data appear to be shaped roughly like a bell-shaped curve
Null hypothesis	A negative hypothesis regarding an experimental result among an underlying population of interest
Number needed to treat/harm	1/absolute value(attributable risk) The number of people who would need to be treated to prevent a single occurrence of an outcome
Observational study	A type of study design in which the investigators observe exposures that occur naturally. Observational studies include case series, cross-sectional studies, cohort studies, and case-control studies
Odds ratio	A ratio of the odds of disease among exposed persons to the odds of disease among unexposed persons. The odds ratio is the principal measure of risk in case-control studies
Outcome	The characteristic that is being predicted in a study
Outlier	A data point that resides far away from most of the other data
Percent agreement	(Number of tests that agree/total number of tests) × 100% Describes the proportion of binary tests that are in agreement between two observers
Per-protocol analysis *As-treated analysis*	Evaluates participants according to the interventions that they actually received during a trial. Subject to bias
Person-time	The summation of study time contributed by a unified group of people, such as a cohort. Used for calculating incidence rates
Pharmacoepidemiology studies	Observational studies of the consequences of medications or procedures
Phase I studies	Studies that administer a new drug to a small group of volunteers to understand how well the drug is tolerated
Phase II studies	Studies that assess the biologic activity of a new drug based on effects on biologic markers and surrogate endpoints
Phase III studies	Randomized clinical trials designed to determine the impact of a new drug on clinically relevant outcomes
Phase IV studies	Studies of real-world drug effectiveness typically conducted after regulatory approval
Placebo	A substance or procedure that is perceived as therapy but has no biologic or therapeutic activity
Population	All people in the world or universe who fit some particular description. Typically, the population refers to all people who are similar to the participants in a research study

Population attributable risk	Incidence(total population) – Incidence(unexposed cohort) Describes the quantity of additional outcomes in the study population that is presumably due to the exposure
Population attributable risk %	$$\frac{\left[\text{Incidence}\left(\text{total population}\right) - \text{Incidence}\left(\text{unexposed cohort}\right)\right] \times 100\%}{\text{Incidence}\left(\text{total population}\right)}$$
Positive predictive value	$$\frac{\text{Number of people with gold} - \text{standard disease who test positive}}{\text{Number of people who test positive}}$$ The probability of having actual disease given a positive test
Power	The ability of a statistical test to detect some pre-specified difference or effect. Specifically, power is the probability that a particular study will *not* make a type II error, given an assumption about the difference in a characteristic among groups
Pragmatic study	Studies that assess the practical impact of treatments or risk factors among diverse groups of people in realistic settings
Pretest probability of disease	The expected chance of disease in a person before administering a test. For screening tests, pretest probability is the prevalence of the disease in the underlying population. For diagnostic tests, pretest probability is the suspected chance of the disease based on the clinical presentation.
Precision *Reliability*; *repeatability*	The ability of a test or measurement to return the same result when performed in succession
Predictor variable	A variable in a regression model used to predict the outcome variable. Typically, a predictor variable is a treatment or exposure
Prevalence *Point prevalence* *Period prevalence*	Prevalence of disease = Incidence of disease × duration of the disease The amount of a disease that is present in a population at a specific time point or during a specific time period
Prevalent disease	A past history of a chronic condition. Typically used to describe diseases that may be treated but are rarely cured
Prevalent user bias	A type of bias that can occur in studies that preferentially evaluate long-standing users of a particular medication
Primary prevention	The administration of treatments intended to prevent the initial occurrence of disease among people without evidence of the disease
Propensity score matching	A method used to control for confounding in which a statistical model estimates the likelihood of the study exposure based on multiple participant characteristics
Prospective study	A descriptive term used to describe studies that are conceived before the data are collected
Quantiles *Percentiles*	Specific values within a distribution that divide the data into groups. Examples of quantiles include tertiles (three equally sized groups) and quartiles (four equally sized groups)
Quantitative outcomes	Continuous study outcome measurements, such as systolic blood pressure, tumor size, or weight
Random assignment *Randomization*	A procedure used in interventional studies to increase the degree of similarity in participant characteristics across treatment groups

Randomized trial *Randomized study*	A type of interventional study that uses a random procedure to assign participants to one or more treatment or control groups
Recall bias *Information bias* *Differential misclassification*	A type of bias that can arise in case-control studies due to differential recall of previous exposures between people who have a disease and those who do not. Recall bias is a type of differential misclassification of the exposure
Receiver operating characteristic (ROC) curve	A graphical description of the sensitivity and specificity values for all possible choices of a cutoff value for a continuous test
Reference cohort	A designated unexposed cohort that serves as the comparator for other study cohorts
Referral bias	A type of bas that can occur in observational studies of screening in which differences between screened and unscreened people confound the association of the screening procedure with study outcomes
Regression	A mathematical method used to describe the relationship, or association, between two or more study variables
Relative risk	Incidence(exposed cohort)/Incidence(unexposed cohort) The relative probability of disease comparing exposed or treated individuals to unexposed or untreated individuals.
Reliability *Repeatability*; *precision*	The ability of a test or measurement to return the same result when performed in succession
Residual	The difference between the value predicted from a regression equation and the actual observed value
Residual confounding	Confounding due to characteristics that are not measured in a study, or characteristics that are measured inaccurately
Restricted randomization	Procedures used in randomized trials to increase the degree of similarity among the intervention groups. Examples include *block randomization* and *stratified randomization*
Restriction	A method used to control for confounding by removing all participants who have a particular characteristic of interest
Retrospective study	A descriptive term used to describe studies that are conducted after the data have been collected
Reverse causality	A type of bias that can occur when the outcome of a study influences the level of the exposure. Cross-sectional studies are most susceptible to this problem
Run-in period	A planned stage of a trial conducted prior to randomization to assess compliance, reduce the possibility of harm, or identify suitable people for subsequent randomization
Sample	A subset of a given population. A sample in the context of a research study typically refers to the study population (which is actually *not* a population)
Sample size	The number of people in a research study
Scatter plot	A graph plotting the raw values of two characteristics
Screening	Testing for disease during the preclinical phase, in which the disease has not yet caused recognizable signs or symptoms
Secondary prevention	The administration of treatments intended to prevent the occurrence of disease among people who have subclinical disease detected by screening

Sensitivity	$$\frac{\text{Number of people with gold} - \text{standard disease who test positive}}{\text{Number of people with gold} - \text{standard disease}}$$
	The proportion of people who test positive among all people with gold-standard evidence of a disease
Significance level	The threshold p-value used to declare statistical significance. Typically set at 0.05
Single blind study	A study in which the participants are unaware of which intervention they are receiving
Simple randomization	Procedures that perform randomization without regard to previous treatment assignments, such as flipping a coin
Skew	The degree of asymmetry in a distribution. Highly skewed distributions do *not* follow a normal, or bell-shaped appearance
Source population	The general setting from which study participants are selected, such as clinics, hospitals, or communities
Specificity	$$\frac{\text{Number with gold} - \text{standard absence of disease who test negative}}{\text{Number with gold} - \text{standard absence of disease}}$$
	The proportion of people who test negative among all people with gold-standard evidence for the absence of a disease
Standard deviation	A common measure of spread, defined as $\sqrt{\text{(variance)}}$
Statistical inference	A process to infer a characteristic of interest in an underlying population based on the results obtained in a sample
Stratification	The process of dividing a population into smaller groups according to a specific characteristic
Stratification plus adjustment	A method used to control for confounding by dividing a study population into smaller groups according to a confounding characteristic and then rejoining these groups after analysis
Stratified randomization	A restricted randomization strategy that performs randomization within pre-specified groups in a clinical trial
Study hypothesis *Alternate hypothesis*	An affirmative hypothesis regarding an experimental result among an underlying population of interest
Study population *Patient population*	All people who enter a study regardless of whether they are treated, develop the disease, or drop out after the study begins
Subclinical disease	Early, clinically silent stages of a disease process. Often requires specialized testing for detection
Subgroup	A smaller group of people within a study population
Subgroup analyses	Analyses performed to explore whether the association of interest differs among smaller groups of participants in a study
Sum of squares	A mathematical procedure used to obtain the best fitting regression equation by minimizing the sum of the squared residuals
Summary measure	A compact description of the study data that conveys information about the distribution of one or more variables quickly
Summary relative risk	A combined relative risk calculated from stratified study data

Surrogate endpoint	A substitute for direct measurements of how a patient feels, functions, or survives. Ideal surrogate endpoints are those that change in response to treatment in a manner consistent with the clinical benefits and harms of the treatment
Survivor function *Kaplan-Meier estimator*	A function, $S(t)$, that returns the cumulative probability of being free of the study outcome at a particular time, t
Synergy	A mutual interaction between two or more risk factors
Survivorship bias	A type of bias that can occur when studying exclusively long-term survivors of a particular disease
T-test	A statistical test used to compare the mean values of a characteristic between two different groups
Temporal association	Demonstration that a potential risk factor was present before the occurrence of the disease
Tertiary prevention	The administration of treatments that target existing disease to improve complications and outcomes of established disease
Two-sample test	A statistical test that compares the value of a characteristic of interest between two different groups
Type I error	A hypothesis test declares a result to be statistically significant when the null hypothesis is actually true (no actual difference in the population)
Type II error	A hypothesis test declares a result to be statistically nonsignificant when the null hypothesis is actually false (actual difference in the population)
Regression	A mathematical procedure used to describe the association between two or more study variables
Regression model *Regression equation*	A mathematical equation fit to the study data
Univariate statistic	A summary measure that pertains to a single study variable
Validity *Accuracy*	The ability of a test or measurement to obtain the true value of the characteristic being measured. In the context of screening and diagnostic testing, validity refers to the ability of a test to identify actual disease, determined by a gold-standard method
Variance *Variation*	A common measure of spread, defined as $\sum (\mu - x_i)^2 / N$ The square root of the variance is the standard deviation
Washout period	An intervening period typically used in crossover trials to separate the effects of different study interventions

Index

© Springer Nature Switzerland AG 2019
B. Kestenbaum, *Epidemiology and Biostatistics*,
https://doi.org/10.1007/978-3-319-96644-1